CALCULATIONS
FOR
VETERINARY
PROFESSIONAL

Moulton, No.

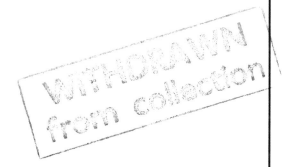

CALCULATIONS FOR THE VETERINARY PROFESSIONAL

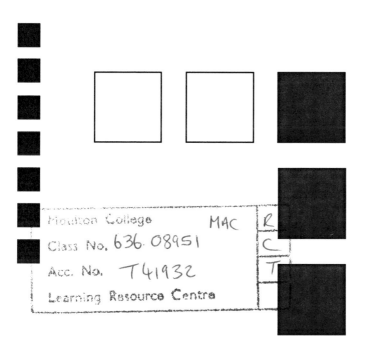

REVISED EDITION

By Vicki C. McConnell, PharmD

Edited by Branson W. Ritchie, DVM, PhD,
Diplomate, ABVP and ECAMS

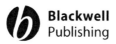

Blackwell
Publishing

Vicki C. McConnell received her BS in Pharmacy from the University of Georgia. She also received her PharmD from the University of Georgia in conjunction with the Medical College of Georgia. She was on staff at the College of Veterinary Medicine, University of Georgia, for nine years. She is a member of the Society of Veterinary Hospital Pharmacists. She is currently working for Florida Hospital Home Infusion, LLP as a consultant and service provider.

Branson W. Ritchie, DVM, PhD, Diplomate, ABVP and ECAMS, is a distinguished research professor in the Department of Small Animal Medicine, College of Veterinary Medicine, University of Georgia.

© 2001 Iowa State University Press
A Blackwell Science Company
All rights reserved

Blackwell Publishing Professional
2121 State Avenue, Ames, Iowa 50014

Orders: 1-800-862-6657
Office: 1-515-292-0140
Fax: 1-515-292-3348
Web site: www.blackwellprofessional.com

Book and cover design: Matthew R. Taets

Authorization to photocopy items for internal or personal use, or the internal or personal use of specific clients, is granted by Blackwell Publishing, provided that the base fee of $.10 per copy is paid directly to the Copyright Clearance Center, 222 Rosewood Drive, Danvers, MA 01923. For those organizations that have been granted a photocopy license by CCC, a separate system of payments has been arranged. The fee code for users of the Transactional Reporting Service is 0-8138-0879-0/2001 $.10.

Ⓧ Printed on acid-free paper in the United States of America

First revised edition, 2001

Library of Congress Cataloging-in-Publication Data

McConnell, Vicki C.
    Calculations for the veterinary professional / by Vicki C. McConnell; edited by Branson W. Ritchie–1st ed.
    p. cm.
    ISBN 0-8138-0879-0
    1. Veterinary drugs–Dosage. I. Ritchie, Branson W. II. Title.

SF919. M33 1999
636.089'514–dc21   99-047112

The last digit is the number: 9   8   7   6   5   4   3   2

Contents

Preface

Each day, veterinary professionals are faced with the task of administering therapeutic agents and nutritional supplements to a range of animals that may vary in size and structure from fish to horses. Those professionals involved with flock or herd management are frequently required to mix chemicals for use as parasiticides, pesticides, or for disinfecting purposes. This book was written to facilitate the completion of these often complex calculations.

A special thank-you to my editor and friend, Dr. Branson Ritchie, who saw a need and patiently worked with me to fill it. Thanks also to my friends at the University of Georgia's College of Veterinary Medicine, and especially to Dr. Doug Kemp, who gave me the opportunity to practice in this unique environment. I miss you all!

The author, editor, and publisher have attempted to ensure the accuracy of the information contained in this book, but we make no claims as to the efficacy of the treatment modalities that are used in the examples. The dosing information contained in these problems is for the purpose of practice only. Suitable references should be consulted for the most appropriate treatment modalities and dosing information.

CALCULATIONS FOR THE VETERINARY PROFESSIONAL

1

Math Basics
Part 1

Fractions and Decimals

Both fractions and decimals can be used to represent numbers; however, most medications and delivery systems (syringes, fluid pumps, etc.) use decimal numbers. There are two components to a decimal number, the whole number (the number to the left of the decimal point) and the fraction (the number to the right of the decimal point). For example, in the number 20.45, the whole number is 20 and the fraction is .45. To avoid errors, a 0 is placed in the whole number position of simple fractions. For example, the decimal number .66 is written as 0.66 and the decimal number .25 is written as 0.25. Each place to the right of the decimal represents a factor of 10.

For example, in the decimal 0.142, the 1 represents 10ths, the 4 represents 100ths, and the 2 represents 1000ths.

These numbers can be expressed in another way: tenths (1/10), hundredths (4/100), thousandths (2/1000). Thus:

$$1/10 = 0.1$$
$$4/100 = 0.04$$
$$2/1000 = 0.002$$

Decimal numbers are added, subtracted, multiplied, and divided just like any other number.

```
   0.24
   0.3
+  0.06
──────
   0.6
```

```
   0.77
−  0.21
−  0.08
──────
   0.48
```

0.12 ÷ 0.34 ≈ 0.35
0.27 × 0.79 × 0.61 ≈ 0.13

If necessary, a decimal number can be converted to a fraction by using the number in the numerator and choosing the correct denominator. For example, 0.3 can be converted to 3/10 and 0.25 can be converted to 25/100. In the latter example, 25/100 can be reduced to its simplest term by dividing the numerator and denominator by 25. Thus, 25 ÷ 25 = 1 and 100 ÷ 25 = 4; so 25/100 = 1/4.

To convert any fraction to its decimal equivalent, divide the numerator (top number in a fraction) by the denominator (bottom number in a fraction). For example, to convert the fraction 1/4 to its decimal equivalent, the numerator (1) is divided by the denominator (4): (1 ÷ 4 = 0.25). This same procedure can be used to convert any fraction to its decimal equivalent. Once fractions have been converted to decimals, the resulting number can be easily inserted into any calculation.

★ **Example**: *Multiply 3/5 by 1/2.*
Convert 3/5 to a decimal number by dividing 3 by 5: (3 ÷ 5 = 0.6).
Convert 1/2 to a decimal number by dividing 1 by 2: (1 ÷ 2 = 0.5).
Now, multiply 0.6 × 0.5 = 0.3.

★ **Example**: *Divide 2/5 by 7/9. This also can be written as (2/5)/(7/9).*
Convert 2/5 to a decimal number by dividing 2 by 5: (2 ÷ 5 = 0.4).
Convert 7/9 to a decimal number by dividing 7 by 9: (7 ÷ 9: = 0.77).
Now divide 0.4 by 0.77: (0.4 ÷ 0.77 = 0.52).

Fractions greater than 1 (those that contain a whole number and a fraction like 2 1/5) also can be converted to their decimal equivalent. This conversion is accomplished by changing the fraction to a decimal number followed by adding the two numbers together.

★ **Example:** *Convert 2 1/5 to its decimal equivalent. First, convert 1/5 to a decimal number by dividing 1 by 5: (1 ÷ 5 = 0.2). Now add 2 + 0.2 to get 2.2.*

★ **Example:** *Convert 18 9/20 to its decimal equivalent. First, convert 9/20 to a decimal number by dividing 9 by 20: (9 ÷ 20 = 0.45). Now add 18 + 0.45 to get 18.45.*

Practice Problems
(See Appendix H for answers)

Convert the following fractions to decimals.

1. 1/2
2. 4/9
3. 3/7
4. 9/10
5. 1/15

6. 4/10
7. 2/3
8. 5/8
9. 21/50
10. 75/100

Perform the following calculations:

	Adding decimals	Subtracting decimals	Multiplying decimals	Dividing decimals
11.	0.11 + 2.45	9.04 − 0.2	0.11 × 2.45	9.04 ÷ 0.2
12.	0.23 + 0.71	0.01 − 0.003	0.23 × 0.71	0.01 ÷ 0.003
13.	10.45 + 2.37	2.6 − 1.4	10.45 × 2.37	2.6 ÷ 1.4
14.	0.05 + 0.12	5.03 − 0.06	0.05 × 0.12	5.03 ÷ 0.06
15.	0.001 + 0.02	0.34 − 0.22	0.01 × 0.2	0.34 ÷ 0.22
16.	3.4 + 1.2	1.7 − 0.5	3.4 × 1.2	1.7 ÷ 0.5
17.	0.02 + 0.002	0.003 − 0.001	0.02 × 0.02	0.003 ÷ 0.001
18.	1.1 + 0.6	3.4 − 1.06	1.1 × 0.6	3.4 ÷ 1.06
19.	3.04 + 0.5	14.2 − 3.07	3.04 × 0.05	14.2 ÷ 3.07
20.	6.14 + 2.7	6.88 − 0.12	6.14 × 2.7	6.88 ÷ 0.12

Scientific Notation

Large numbers are often written using scientific notation to make their manipulation easier. Exponential notation is a way to express any number (b) as a coefficient (n) times the power of 10. For example, the number 28,967,345 can be converted to the scientific number 2.8967345×10^7. A scientific number can be converted to its original number by moving the decimal point to the right (if positive) or to the left (if negative) the correct number of places according to the coefficient. For example, the scientific number 5.467×10^3 can also be expressed as 5,467. Scientific numbers also make it possible to work with numbers that are only a fraction of 1. For example, the number 0.000046 can be written as 4.6×10^{-5}. Note that when a decimal place is moved to the left, the power of 10 is positive (the original number is greater than 1), and when the decimal place is moved to the right, the power of 10 is negative (the original number is less than 1). Thus,

$10^1 = 10$ $\qquad$ $10^{-1} = 0.1$

$10^2 = 100$ $\qquad$ $10^{-2} = 0.01$

$10^3 = 1000$ $\qquad$ $10^{-3} = 0.001$

$10^4 = 10,000$ $\qquad$ $10^{-4} = 0.0001$

$10^5 = 100,000$ $\qquad$ $10^{-5} = 0.00001$

$10^6 = 1,000,000$ $\qquad$ $10^{-6} = 0.000001$

$10^7 = 10,000,000$ $\qquad$ $10^{-7} = 0.0000001$

$10^8 = 100,000,000$ $\qquad$ $10^{-8} = 0.00000001$

Logarithms (Log)

Logarithm is defined as the power to which a selected base (b) must be raised in order to equal the number y:

$y = b^n$, where n is the logarithm of y to base b (written as $\log_b x$).

In common logarithms, every number may be expressed as a power of 10. The exponent is the number that indicates what power of 10 must be raised to equal a given number.

In natural logarithms, unlike common logs, natural or Naperian logs have a base number.

$\log 1 = 0$	$\log 0.1 = -1$
$\log 10 = 1$	$\log 0.01 = -2$
$\log 100 = 2$	$\log 0.001 = -3$
$\log 1000 = 3$	$\log 0.0001 = -4$
$\log 10,000 = 4$	$\log 0.00001 = -5$
$\log 100,000 = 5$	$\log 0.000001 = -6$

Ratios and Proportions

Ratios

It is common to encounter situations in which a dose is listed in one system of measurement and a drug's concentration is given in different units or even in a different system of measurement. For example, a dose may be given in milligrams per kilogram (mg/kg) and the drug may be available in tablets that are provided in grains (gr). To simplify conversions between different systems of measurement, a chart has been provided with common conversions (See Appendix G). Converting between units and or systems of measure can also be accomplished using the principle of ratios. A *ratio* is a mathematical expression of a relationship between two different groups of numbers. In most cases, ratios are expressed as fractions and their cross products are equal to each other. That is, the value is obtained when the numerator (number on the top) of the first number is multiplied by the denominator (number on the bottom) of the second number, as in the example below:

$$\frac{2}{7} \times \frac{8}{23}$$

By cross multiplying,

$$2 \times 23 = 7 \times 8$$

$$56 = 56$$

The units on the numerator (number on top) and denominator (number on bottom) can be the same:

$$\frac{\text{lower percent concentration}}{\text{larger percent concentration}} = \frac{\text{lower volume}}{\text{larger volume}}$$

or they can be different:

$$\frac{\text{mg}}{\text{ml}} = \frac{\text{mg}}{\text{ml}}$$

When cross multiplied the units on each side should be equal:

$$\frac{\text{lower percent concentration}}{\text{larger percent concentration}} = \frac{\text{lower volume}}{\text{larger volume}}$$

concentration × volume = concentration × volume
or

$$\frac{\text{mg}}{\text{ml}} = \frac{\text{mg}}{\text{ml}}$$

mg × ml = mg × ml

★ **Example:** *A patient is to receive 30 mEq of potassium chloride. The drug is available in a solution containing 40 mEq/20 ml. How many milliliters of the solution should the patient receive?*

$$\frac{\text{lower percent concentration}}{\text{larger percent concentration}} = \frac{\text{lower volume}}{\text{larger volume}}$$

$$\frac{30 \text{ mEq}}{40 \text{ mEq}} = \frac{\text{unknown ml}}{20 \text{ ml}}$$

Cross multiply to solve the equation:

unknown ml × 40 mEq = 30 mEq × 20 ml

$$\text{unknown ml} = \frac{30 \text{ mEq} \times 20 \text{ ml}}{40 \text{ mEq}}$$

unknown ml = **15 ml**

★ **Example:** *A snake is referred that has been receiving 2 ml of injectable penicillin G (200,000 U/ml). How many units of penicillin G did the snake receive with each dose?*

$$\frac{1 \text{ ml}}{2 \text{ ml}} = \frac{200,000 \text{ U}}{\text{unknown U}}$$

Cross multiply to solve the equation:

unknown U × 1 ml = 200,000 U × 2 ml

$$\text{unknown U} = \frac{200,000 \text{ U}}{1 \text{ ml}} \times 2 \text{ ml}$$

unknown U = **400,000 U**

★ **Example:** *A cat is prescribed 40 mg of aspirin to control pain following surgery. Aspirin is available in 1 1/4 and 5 grain tablets. a) How many milligrams of aspirin are in a 1 1/4 gr tablet? b) How many tablets will the cat need?*

a) Grains can be converted to milligrams using the conversion tables in Appendix G:

1 grain = 64.8 mg

1.25 ~~grain aspirin~~ × 64.8 mg/~~grain~~ = 81 mg

Thus a 1 1/4 grain tablet contains 81 mg of aspirin. Alternately, a ratio can be used to convert from grains to milligrams using the fact that 1 grain = 64.8 mg:

$$\frac{1 \text{ gr}}{64.8 \text{ mg}} = \frac{1.25 \text{ gr}}{\text{unknown mg}}$$

Cross multiply to solve the equation:

1 gr × unknown mg = 1.25 gr × 64.8 mg

$$\text{unknown mg} = \frac{1.25 \text{ ~~gr~~} \times 64.8 \text{ mg}}{1 \text{ ~~gr~~}}$$

unknown mg = **81 mg**

b) To determine the number of tablets the cat will require, take the milligram dose required and divide it by the strength of the tablet in milligrams:

$$\text{tablets needed} = \frac{\text{dose (mg)}}{\text{table strength}}$$

$$\text{tablets needed} = \frac{40 \text{ mg}}{81 \text{ mg per tablet}}$$

tablets needed ≈ **0.5 tablet**

★ **Example:** *An anorectic dog is to be fed via a feeding tube. If the dog is to receive 150 ml total volume of food mixture diluted 1:3 in water three times a day, how much food and how much water will the dog need?*

$$\frac{\text{lower percent concentration}}{\text{larger percent concentration}} = \frac{\text{lower volume}}{\text{larger volume}}$$

$$\frac{1 \text{ part food}}{4 \text{ parts total}} = \frac{\text{unknown ml}}{150 \text{ ml mixture}}$$

Cross multiply to solve the equation:

1 part food × 150 ml = unknown ml × 4 parts total

$$\text{unknown ml} = \frac{1 \times 150}{4}$$

unknown ml = **37.5 ml of food**

If 150 ml contains 37.5 ml food, then 112.5 ml of water will be added for each feeding. This amount of water is obtained by subtracting the amount of food from the total amount given (150 ml – 37.5 ml = 112.5 ml water).

★ **Example:** *A bird needs 200 mg of ticarcillin. The vial of lypholized ticarcillin gives instructions to add 18.5 ml of diluent to make a 0.155 g/ml solution. How many milliliters of the stock preparation will be needed to give the bird the required 200 mg?*

Step 1:
Convert from grams per milliliter to milligrams per milliliter using the fact that
1 g = 1000 mg:

$$\frac{0.155 \text{ g}}{\text{ml}} \times \frac{1000 \text{ mg}}{\text{g}} = 155 \text{ mg / ml}$$

Step 2:
Solve for the volume of ticarcillin required to provide 200 mg using the ratio:

$$\frac{\text{amount of drug needed}}{\text{concentration available}} = \frac{\text{unknown volume to give}}{\text{known volume of drug}}$$

$$\frac{200 \text{ mg}}{155 \text{ mg}} = \frac{\text{unknown ml}}{1}$$

Cross multiply to solve the equation:

unknown volume to give × 155 = 1 × 200

$$\text{unknown volume to give} = \frac{200}{155}$$

volume to give = **1.29 ml**

★ **Example:** *A dog is to receive 10 units of U-100 insulin. How many milliliters will be needed? (U-100 insulin contains 100 units of insulin per milliliter).*

$$\frac{\text{amount of drug needed}}{\text{concentration available}} = \frac{\text{unknown ml to give}}{\text{known volume of drug}}$$

$$\frac{10 \text{ units}}{100 \text{ units}} = \frac{\text{unknown ml}}{1 \text{ ml}}$$

Cross multiply to solve the equation:

100 U × unknown ml = 10 U

$$\text{unknown ml} = \frac{10 \text{ U}}{100 \text{ U}}$$

ml to give = **0.1 ml**

Proportions

A proportion is the expression of the equality of two ratios such as

$a:b = c:d$ or $\dfrac{a}{b} = \dfrac{c}{d}$

★ **Example:** *If 2 tablets of aspirin contain 10 grains, how many grains are in 10 tablets?*

Set up a proportion like this:

$$\frac{10 \text{ grains}}{2 \text{ tablets}} = \frac{\text{unknown grains}}{10 \text{ tablets}}$$

Cross mulitply to solve the equation:

unknown grains × 2 tablets = 10 grains × 10 tablets

unknown grains $= \dfrac{100}{2}$

Grains in 10 tablets = **50 grains**

★ **Example:** *If 5 ml of Amoxidrops® contains 250 mg, how many milliliters are needed for a dose of 350 mg?*

$$\frac{250 \text{ mg}}{5 \text{ ml}} = \frac{350 \text{ mg}}{\text{unknown ml}}$$

Cross multiply to solve the equation:

unknown ml × 250 mg = 5 ml × 350 mg

unknown ml $= \dfrac{5 \text{ ml} \times 350 \text{ mg}}{250 \text{ mg}}$

volume of Amoxidrops = **7 ml**

★ **Example:** *If epinephrine is available as a 1:10,000 solution, a) what is the concentration in mg/ml, b) what is the percentage, and c) how many ml are required to give a dose of 5 mg?*

a) By convention, a 1:10,000 solution contains 1 g/10,000 ml. Convert from grams to milligrams using the fact that 1 gram is equal to 1000 mg (See Appendix G):

$$\text{concentration} = \frac{1\ \cancel{g}}{10,000\ \text{ml}} \times \frac{1000\ \text{mg}}{1\ \cancel{g}}$$

$$\text{concentration} = \frac{1 \times 1000\ \text{mg}}{10,000\ \text{ml}}$$

$$\text{concentration} = \frac{1000\ \text{mg}}{10,000\ \text{ml}}$$

concentration = **0.1 mg/ml**

b) A drug concentration may be expressed as a percentage, which is equal to the number of grams of drug contained in 100 ml of solution.
That is,

concentration% = concentration in g/100 ml.

Step 1:
Convert epinephrine's concentration from milligrams per milliliter to grams per milliliter:

$$\text{concentration} = \frac{0.1\ \cancel{\text{mg}}}{\text{ml}} \times \frac{1\ \text{g}}{1000\ \cancel{\text{mg}}}$$

$$\text{concentration} = \frac{0.1\ \text{g}}{1000\ \text{ml}}$$

concentration = 0.0001 g/ml

Step 2:
Set up a ratio to determine the number of grams contained in 100 milliliters:

$$\frac{0.0001 \text{ g}}{1 \text{ ml}} = \frac{\text{unknown g}}{100 \text{ ml}}$$

Cross multiply to solve the equation:
unknown g × 1 g = 0.0001 g × 100 ml

$$\text{unknown g} = \frac{0.01 \text{ g}}{1 \text{ ml}} = 0.01 \text{ g/ml}$$

concentration by % = **0.01%**

Alternate Method:
The concentration could also have been determined in milligrams per 100 milliliters:

$$\frac{0.1 \text{ mg}}{1 \text{ ml}} = \frac{\text{unknown mg}}{100 \text{ ml}}$$

Cross multiply to solve the equation:
unknown concentration = 0.1 mg × 100 ml

$$\text{unknown concentration} = \frac{10 \text{ mg}}{100 \text{ ml}}$$

and then convert to g/100 ml = %:

$$\text{concentration} = \frac{10 \; \cancel{\text{mg}}}{100 \text{ ml}} \times \frac{1 \text{ g}}{1000 \; \cancel{\text{mg}}}$$

$$\text{concentration} = \frac{10 \text{ g}}{100,000 \text{ ml}}$$

Divide numerator and denominator by 1000 to convert to 100 milliliters:

$$\text{concentration} = \frac{10 \text{ g}}{100,000 \text{ ml}} \div \frac{1000}{1000}$$

$$\text{concentration} = \frac{0.01 \text{ g}}{100 \text{ ml}}$$

concentration by % = **0.01%**

c) To determine the number of milliliters required to deliver a 5 mg dose, recall that

$$0.01\% = \frac{0.01 \text{ g}}{100 \text{ ml}} = \frac{10 \text{ mg}}{100 \text{ ml}} = \frac{0.1 \text{ mg}}{\text{ml}}$$

and set up a ratio:

$$\frac{0.1 \text{ mg}}{1 \text{ ml}} = \frac{5 \text{ mg}}{\text{unknown ml}}$$

Cross multiply to solve the equation:

unknown ml × 0.1 = 5

$$\text{unknown ml} = \frac{5}{0.1}$$

volume to give = **50 ml**

Practice Problems
(See Appendix H for answers)

21. How much 0.2 mg/ml Dilaudid® solution can be made from 2 ml of 10 mg/ml Dilaudid®?

22. What volume of 0.25% phenylephrine solution can be prepared from 5 ml of 2% phenylephrine solution?

23. How much 50 mg/ml morphine sulfate solution can be prepared using ten 30 mg morphine sulfate soluble tablets?

24. How long will it take to infuse a 1 g dose of Dilantin® at a rate of 50 mg/minute?

25. If household bleach (5% sodium hypochlorite) is diluted 1:32, what is the final concentration of sodium hypochlorite?

Temperature

Temperature can be measured using a variety of scales. The Fahrenheit scale (°F) was commonly used in the United States in the 20th century. In an attempt to standardize units of weight and measure, the metric system is used more today, where temperature is expressed in Celsius (°C). Scientists working with very cold conditions measure temperature in degrees Kelvin (°K). Learning to convert between these scales can prove valuable in assessing the proper storage condition of labortory samples and medications as well as in determining body temperature.

Conversion Equations
from Fahrenheit to Celsius: °C = (°F − 32) × 5/9
from Celsius to Fahrenheit: °F = (9/5 × °C) + 32
from Celsius to Kelvin: °K = °C + 273
from Kelvin to Celsius: °C = °K − 273
from Fahrenheit to Kelvin: °K = (°F − 32) × 9/5 + 273
from Kelvin to Fahrenheit: °F = 9/5 (°K − 273) + 32

★ **Example:** *If a laboratory sample is to be chilled to 2°C, what is the temperature in °F?*

Temperature conversion from Celsius to Fahrenheit:

°F = (9/5 × °C) + 32
°F = (9/5 × 2) + 32
°F = 18/5 + 32
°F = **35.6°**

★ **Example:** *If a dog's temperature is 101.5°F, what is its temperature in °C?*

Temperature conversion from Fahrenheit to Celsius:

°C = (°F − 32) × 5/9
°C = (101.5 − 32) × 5/9
°C = 69.5 × 5/9
°C = 38.6°

★ **Example:** *If a bird's normal temperature is 103.5°F, what is its temperature in °C?*

Temperature conversion from Fahrenheit to Celsius:

°C = (°F − 32) × 5/9
°C = (103.5° − 32) × 5/9
°C = 39.72°

★ **Example:** *If a temperature is −63°C, what is the corresponding temperature in °K?*

Temperature conversion from Celsius to Kelvin:

°K = °C + 273
°K = − 63° + 273
°K = 210°

Practice Problems
(See Appendix H for answers)

26. If the outside temperature is 21°C, what is the temperature in °F?
27. Water freezes at 32°F, so what is the corresponding temperature in °C?
28. Water boils at 212°F, so what is the corresponding temperature in °C?
29. If a water bath needs to be 9°C, what is the corresponding temperature in °F?
30. If a freezer is −27°C, what is the temperature in°K?

Units

Some drugs in the veterinary community are available in United States Pharmacopoeia (USP) Units or International Units (IU). A "U" indicates the number of units of an agent per ml. For example, 1 ml of U-100 insulin contains 100 units of insulin. Stated another way, 10,000 U heparin means 10,000 units of heparin per milliliter.

Converting Units to Milliliters

To determine the quantity of drug required in milliliters when the product available is in units, use the equation:

$$\frac{\text{required dose (units)}}{\text{drug amount (ml)}} = \frac{\text{concentration available (units)}}{1 \text{ ml}}$$

★ **Example:** *It is determined that a dog with polydipsia, polyuria, and liver disease is diabetic. The dog weighs 27 lb and needs 5 units of insulin per day. How many milliliters of U-100 insulin will be needed?*

$$\frac{\text{required dose (units)}}{\text{drug amount (ml)}} = \frac{\text{concentration available (units)}}{1 \text{ ml}}$$

$$\frac{5 \text{ U}}{\text{unknown ml}} = \frac{100 \text{ U}}{1 \text{ ml}}$$

Cross multiply to solve the equation:

unknown ml × 100 U = 5 U × 1 ml

$$\text{unknown ml} = \frac{5 \cancel{U} \times 1 \text{ ml}}{100 \cancel{U}}$$

insulin volume = **0.05 ml**

★ **Example:** *As part of anticoagulative therapy for a saddle thrombus, a cat is to receive 1,500 units of heparin intravenously. The heparin is available in a 10,000 U/ml solution. How many milliliters of the solution should the cat receive?*

$$\frac{\text{required dose (units)}}{\text{drug amount (ml)}} = \frac{\text{concentration available (units)}}{1 \text{ ml}}$$

$$\frac{\text{unknown ml}}{1,500 \text{ U}} = \frac{1 \text{ ml}}{10,000 \text{ U}}$$

Cross multiply to solve the equation:

unknown ml × 10,000 U = 1 ml × 1,500 U

$$\text{unknown ml} = \frac{1,500 \text{ ml}}{10,000}$$

heparin volume = **0.15 ml**

★ **Example:** *You run out of U-1000 heparin flush. How much 20,000 U/ml heparin is needed to make 100 ml of a 1000 U/ml solution?*

Determine the total amount of heparin (in units) required by multiplying the volume needed (100 ml) by the concentration desired (1000 U/ml).

100 ml × 1,000 U/ml = 100,000 U

Then, set up the equation as before:

$$\frac{\text{required dose (units)}}{\text{drug amount (ml)}} = \frac{\text{concentration available (units)}}{1 \text{ ml}}$$

$$\frac{100,000 \text{ U}}{\text{unknown ml}} = \frac{20,000 \text{ U}}{1 \text{ ml}}$$

Cross multiply to solve the equation:

unknown ml × 20,000 U = 100,000 U × 1 ml

$$\text{unknown ml} = \frac{100,000 \, \cancel{U} \times 1 \text{ ml}}{20,000 \, \cancel{U}}$$

volume needed = **5 ml**

Alternatively, this problem can be solved by

initial conc × initial volume = final conc × final volume

20,000 U × unknown ml = 1000 U × 100 ml

$$\text{unknown ml} = \frac{1000 \, \cancel{U} \times 100 \text{ ml}}{20,000 \, \cancel{U}}$$

volume needed = **5 ml**

Thus, to make 100 ml of 1000 U/ml heparin flush, dilute 5 ml of 20,000 U/ml heparin in 95 ml of 0.9% sodium chloride.

★ **Example:** *A 70 lb dog is being treated with heparin for DIC at a dose of 150 U/kg. You have 1000 U/ml sodium heparin in the pharmacy. How many ml are needed per dose?*

Step 1:
Using the fact that 1 kg = 2.2 lb, convert the weight of the animal from pounds to kilograms:
(See Appendix G):

Set up a ratio:

$$\frac{\text{unknown kg}}{70 \text{ lb}} = \frac{1 \text{ kg}}{2.2 \text{ lb}}$$

Cross multiply to solve the equation:

unknown kg × 2.2 lb = 70 lb × 1 kg

$$\text{unknown kg} = \frac{70 \cancel{\text{lb}} \times 1 \text{ kg}}{2.2 \cancel{\text{lb}}}$$

unknown kg = 32 kg

Step 2:
Now determine the total dose needed:

dose needed = 32 kg × 150 U / kg

dose needed = 4,800 U

What If There Is an Overdose?

★ **Example:** *The dog in the previous example accidentally received 10 ml of heparin. Protamine is listed in your formulary as the antidote for heparin overdose. One mg of protamine neutralizes 90 USP units of sodium heparin derived from the lung or 115 USP units heparin derived from intestinal mucosa. The heparin you stock is derived from beef lung according to the bottle. How much protamine is needed to reverse the excess heparin given?*

Step 1:
Calculate the amount of excess heparin received:

excess heparin = heparin received − calculated dose

excess heparin = 1000 U/ml × 10 ml − 4,800 U

excess heparin = 5,200 U

Step 2:
Divide the dose of excess heparin by the activity of protamine (1 mg/90 U) to determine the amount of protamine required:

$$\text{protamine required} = 5{,}200 \; \cancel{\text{U heparin}} \times \frac{1 \text{ mg protamine}}{90 \; \cancel{\text{U heparin}}}$$

protamine required = **58.1 mg**

Converting between Units and Milligrams

By convention:
1 USP unit vit D = 1 IU vit D = 0.025 mcg vit D_3
1 mg vit D_3 = 40,000 U vit D activity
1.25 mg vit D_2 = 50,000 IU of vit D activity
1 mg DHT= 3 mg vit D_2 = 120, 000 IU vit D activity

★ **Example:** *The dose for DHT (dihydrotachysterol) in dogs is 0.01 mg/kg q24h. If a 30 lb dog needs supplementation for hypocalcemia secondary to hypoparathyroidism, how much DHT should it receive?*

Step 1:
Convert the weight from pounds to kilograms (See Appendix G):

$$\frac{30 \; \cancel{\text{lb}} \times 1 \text{ kg}}{2.2 \; \cancel{\text{lb}}} = 13.6 \text{ kg}$$

Step 2:
Multiply the weight in kilograms by the daily dose:

$$\frac{13.6 \; \cancel{\text{kg}} \times 0.01 \text{ mg}}{1 \; \cancel{\text{kg}} / \text{day}} = 0.136 \text{ mg/day}$$

Step 3:

DHT is available in 0.125 mg tablets and capsules, 0.2 mg and 0.4 mg tablets, and solutions of 0.2 mg/ml and 0.25 mg/ml. You decide to use the oral solution containing 0.25 mg/ml because the intensol solution (0.2 mg/ml) is 20% alcohol. How much of the oral solution do you need?

$$\frac{0.136 \text{ mg}}{1 \text{ day}} \times \frac{1 \text{ ml}}{0.25 \text{ mg}} = 0.54 \text{ ml / day}$$

The solution is available in 15 ml bottles. How many days' supply is in one bottle?

$$\frac{15 \text{ ml}}{0.54 \text{ ml / day}} = 27.7 \text{ days}$$

How many units of vitamin D activity is this dog receiving each day? As stated previously, 1 mg DHT=120,000 U of vitamin D activity. Thus,

$$0.136 \text{ mg DHT} \times \frac{120,000 \text{ U}}{1 \text{ mg DHT}} = 16,320 \text{ U}$$

You have run out of DHT on a Friday. You do have D_2 liquid that contains 8,000 U/ml. How much D_2 liquid do you need to give each day until a new supply of DHT arrives?

$$\frac{16,320 \text{ U}}{1 \text{ day}} \times \frac{1 \text{ ml}}{8,000 \text{ U}} = 2.04 \text{ ml / day}$$

Practice Problems
(See Appendix H for answers)

31. If a dog needs 10,000 units of vitamin D activity each day, how many milligrams of vitamin D_3 are needed?

32. Vitamin E comes in several forms of varying potencies. Dosage is usually standardized in International Units (IU) based on activity. Aquasol E® contains 50 mg/ml as d-alpha tocopheryl actetate. If 1 mg of d-alpha tocopheryl acetate = 1.36 IU of vitamin E, how many International Units of vitamin E are contained in 2 ml of Aquasol E®?

33. How much U-100 heparin is needed to make 10 ml of 10 U/ml heparin flush?

34. If a cat's dose of ultralente insulin is 4 units, what is the volume of U-100 insulin required per dose?

35. What volume of U-100 insulin should be used to make 10 ml of diluted insulin with a final concentration of 10 U/ml?

Volume

The determination of the volume of a container can be beneficial in herd medicine as well as aquaculture. Equations for the common, and not so common, shapes of tanks are given below. See figures in Appendix A under Volume Equations.

Volume Equations

triangular trough = 1/2 [base × height × length]
rectangular trough = length × width × height
cylindrical trough = 3.14 × (radius)^2 × height
truncated cone = 1.05 × h × [(r1)^2 + (r1 × r2) + (r2)^2]

★ **Example:** *Clients have a cylindrical fish tank in their place of business that you wish to treat for ick. The tank is 6 feet tall and 4 feet across. How many gallons of water does the tank hold?*

Step 1:
volume cylindrical trough = 3.14 × (radius)* × height

*radius = diameter / 2

$$\text{radius} = \frac{4}{2} = 2$$

volume = 3.14 × (2 ft)^2 × 6 ft
volume = 3.14 × 4 ft^2 × 6 ft
volume = 75.36 ft^3

Step 2:
To convert the volume of the tank from cubic feet to cubic centimeters (See Appendix G):
1 ft = 12 in.
1 in. = 2.54 cm

$$\text{volume in cm}^3 = 75.36 \text{ ft}^3 \times \left[\frac{2.54 \text{ cm}}{1 \text{ in.}} \times \frac{12 \text{ in.}}{1 \text{ ft}} \right]^3$$

volume in cm^3 = 75.36 × (30.48)^3

Calculation Step:
If you have a scientific calculator with a y^x key:
Enter 30.48.
Press the y^x key.
Enter 3.
Press Equal.
Your answer should be 28,316,845.

If you do not have a scientific calculator, multiply
30.48 × 30.48 × 30.48 = 28,316.845

volume in cm^3 = 75.36 ft^3 × 28,316.845 cm^3/ ft^3
volume = 2,133,957.6 cm^3
1 cm^3 = 1 ml (See Appendix G). Thus,
2,133,957.6 cm^3 = 2,133,957.6 ml

Step 3:
To convert from milliliters to gallons:
1 gal = 3,785 ml

volume in gal $= 2,133,957.6 \text{ ml} \times \dfrac{1 \text{ gal}}{3,785 \text{ ml}}$

volume in gal $\approx$ **564 gal**

★ **Example:** *What is the volume of a cylindrical feeder that is 100 ft tall by 50 ft wide?*

cylindrical trough $= 3.14 \times (\text{radius*})^2 \times$ height

radius = diameter/2

radius $= \dfrac{50}{2} = 25$

volume $= 3.14 \times 625 \text{ ft}^2 \times 100 \text{ ft}$
volume $=$ **196,250 ft³**

★ **Example:** *What is the volume in gallons of a triangular feed trough 4 feet long, 3 feet high, and 2 feet across?*

Step 1:
volume $= 1/2$ [base $\times$ height $\times$ length]
volume $= 1/2 \times$ [2 ft $\times$ 3 ft $\times$ 4 ft]
volume $= 12$ ft³

Step 2:
To determine how many gallons of water this trough will hold, first convert cubic feet to cubic centimeters:

1 ft $=$ 12 in.
1 in. $=$ 2.54 cm

$12 \text{ ft}^3 = 12 \times \left[\dfrac{2.54 \text{ cm}}{1 \text{ in.}} \times \dfrac{12 \text{ in.}}{1 \text{ ft}} \right]^3 = 339,802 \text{ cm}^3$

Step 3:
Convert from cm³ (ml) to gallons recalling that 1 gallon contains 3,785 ml (See Appendix G).

$1 \text{ cm}^3 = 1 \text{ ml}$

$3,785 \text{ ml} = 1 \text{ gallon}$

$$\frac{339,802 \text{ ml} \times 1 \text{ gallon}}{3,785 \text{ ml}} = 89.78 \text{ gallons} \approx 90 \text{ gallons}$$

Practice Problems
(See Appendix H for answers)

36. What is the volume in ml/gal of a pail (truncated cone) if the height = 35 cm, r1 = 15 cm, and r2 = 30 cm?
37. What is the volume, in gallons, of a rectangular trough with dimensions of L = 4 ft, W = 2 ft, and H = 1 ft?
38. How many gallons can a triangular trough hold that is 3 yards long, 3 feet wide, and 2 feet wide?

Physical Chemistry

Moles

Molarity may be used to measure or compare the concentration of two substances whether gas or particles in solution. The term is most commonly used in veterinary medicine when making surgical preparation solutions and occasionally when determining I.V. solution requirements.

A mole is the molecular or atomic weight of a substance in grams (mole = grams/molecular wt). One mole of a substance has the exact same number of atoms or molecules as one mole of any other substance. Thus, 1 mole of Na is equal to 1 mole of Cl.

★ **Example:** *How many moles of water are contained in 1 oz?*

Step 1:

By convention, the density of water is equal to 1 (1 ml of water = 1 g of water). 1 oz is 29.57 ml, but 30 ml is often used for convenience. If we approximate 1 oz of water at 30 ml, then it will weigh 30 g. To determine the molecular weight (mw) of water, recall that water's chemical formula is H_2O. There are 2 hydrogen and 1 oxygen in each mole. The molecular weight of hydrogen is 1.009 and the molecular weight of oxygen is 15.999 (See Appendix D).

Therefore,

mw (H_2O) = (2 × 1.009) + (1 × 15.999) = 18.017 ≈ 18

Step 2:

Substitute the molecular weight (mw) of water (18) into the equation to determine how many moles of water are contained in 1 oz:

$$moles = \frac{g}{mw}$$

$$moles = \frac{30\ g}{18\ mw}$$

moles = **1.67**

Therefore, 1 oz of water contains 1.67 moles.

Practice Problems
(See Appendix H for answers)

39. How many moles of sodium chloride (NaCl) are contained in 10 g of table salt?
40. How many grams of potassium chloride (KCl) are needed to make 2 moles of KCl?
41. If a substance has a molecular weight of 79, how many moles are there in 270 g?

42. How many moles of water are contained in 1 cup?
43. How many moles of water are contained in 1 gallon?

Millimoles

$$\text{millimoles (mm)} = \frac{g \times 1000}{mw} = \frac{mg}{mw}$$

★ **Example:** *Determine how many millimoles of calcium chloride (CaCl$_2$) are contained in 100 grams.*

Step 1:
Calculate the molecular weight of CaCl$_2$
(See Appendix D):

mw (CaCl$_2$) = (1 × mw Ca) + (2 × mw Cl)
mw = (1 × 40.08) + (2 × 35.45)
mw = 110.98

Step 2:
Substitute the molecular weight of CaCl$_2$ (110.98) into the equation (moles = grams divided by the molecular weight) to determine the number of moles contained in 100 g of CaCl$_2$:

$$\text{moles} = \frac{g}{mw}$$

$$\text{moles} = \frac{100 \ \cancel{g}}{110.98 \ (\cancel{g} \ / \ \text{mole})}$$

moles = 0.901

Therefore, 100 g of CaCl$_2$ contain 0.901 moles. The number of millimoles contained in 100 g of CaCl$_2$ can now be determined by using the equation: mmoles = moles × 1000.

mmoles = 1000 × moles
mmoles = 1000 × 0.901
mmoles = **901**

Alternate Method:
Thus, 100 grams of $CaCl_2$ contain 901 millimoles.

These three steps can be combined into a single step as follows:

$$mmoles = \frac{g \times 1000}{mw \ (g \ / \ mole)}$$

$$mmoles = \frac{100 \ \cancel{g} \times 1000}{110.98 \ (\cancel{g} \ / \ mole)}$$

mmoles = **901**

Practice Problems
(See Appendix H for answers)
44. How many mmoles of KCl are contained in 17 g?
45. How many grams of NaCl are needed to make 12 mmoles?
46. How many mmoles of water (H_2O) are in 1 pint?
47. How many grams of HCl are needed to make 8 mmoles?
48. How many mmoles of $CaCl_2$ are contained in 1.5 g?

Milliequivalents

An equivalent is the amount of an ionized substance which has the same electrochemical power as 1 mole of hydrogen ions. A milliequivalent is 1/1000 or 10^{-3} or 0.001 of an equivalent. The milliequivalent is most frequently used as a measurement of ionic concentration in a fluid. Many electrolyte solutions are provided in milliequivalents (mEq). For example, the label for a bag of sodium chloride (NaCl) indicates that each liter contains 154 mEq each of sodium and chloride.

---

milliequivalents (mEq) = mmoles × valence*

$$mEq = \frac{mg \times valence}{mw}$$

or

$$mEq = \frac{mg}{atomic\ wt}$$

$$mEq = \frac{mg}{mw} \times valence$$

valence = charge of the particle

★ **Example:** *Calculate the number of milliequivalents in 100 g of calcium chloride (CaCl$_2$).*

milliequivalents (mEq) = mmoles × valence
From the previous example, we calculated that 100 g of CaCl$_2$ contained 901 mmoles.

mEq = 901 × 1 (See Appendix D)
mEq = **901 mmoles**

Alternate Method:
If we had not calculated the number of moles of CaCl$_2$ in 100 g, we could still solve for the number of milliequivalents using the equations:

mEq = mmoles × valence and

$$mmoles = \frac{g \times 1000}{mw}$$

Thus:

$$mEq = \frac{g \times 1000}{mw} \times valence$$

$$mEq = \frac{100 \text{ g} \times 1000}{110.98} \times 1$$

mEq = 901

Converting Milliequivalents to Milliliters

★ **Example:** *If a Vietnamese potbellied pig weighs 120 lb and needs 2 mEq of NaCl/kg of body weight, how many ml of 0.9% NaCl does it need?*

Step 1:
Convert the weight of the animal from pounds to kilograms:

$$\frac{120 \text{ lb}}{1} \times \frac{1 \text{ kg}}{2.2 \text{ lb}} = 54.5 \text{ kg}$$

Step 2:
Multiply the animal's weight in kilograms by 2mEq/kg to determine the dose of NaCl needed:

mEq NaCl required = wt (kg) × dose (mEq/kg)

mEq NaCl required = 54.5 kg × 2 mEq NaCl/kg

NaCl required = 109 mEq

Step 3:

A 0.9% NaCl solution contains 154 mEq/L. To determine the volume of this solution required, set up a ratio:

$$\frac{154 \text{ mEq}}{1 \text{ L}} = \frac{109 \text{ mEq}}{\text{volume needed}}$$

Cross multiply to solve the equation:

volume × 154 mEq = 109 mEq × 1 L

$$\text{volume} = \frac{109 \text{ } \cancel{\text{mEq}} \times \text{L}}{154 \text{ } \cancel{\text{mEq}}}$$

volume = 0.70779 L

$$\text{volume} = 0.70779 \text{ } \cancel{\text{L}} \times \frac{1000 \text{ ml}}{\cancel{\text{L}}}$$

volume = **708 ml**

Alternate Method:

You could use the mEq equation to solve for the number of grams of NaCl:

$$\text{mEq required} = \frac{g}{mw} \times 1000 \times \text{valence}^*$$

$$109 = \frac{g}{mw} \times 1000 \times \text{valence}$$

mw NaCl = 58.5
valence = 1 (from Appendix D)

$$109 = \frac{g}{58.5} \times 1000 \times 1$$

109 = g × 17.094

$$\frac{109}{17.094} = g$$

g = 6.38 g

Now determine the number of grams of NaCl per liter of 0.9% NaCl:

By definition, $\% = \dfrac{g}{100\ ml}$

$0.9\%\ NaCl = \dfrac{0.9\ g}{100\ ml}$

$0.9\%\ NaCl = \dfrac{0.9\ g}{100\ \cancel{ml}} \times \dfrac{1000\ \cancel{ml}}{1\ L} = 9\ g/L$

Now, determine the volume of 0.9% NaCl solution needed using the ratio:

$\dfrac{9\ g}{1\ L} = \dfrac{6.38\ g}{vol\ in\ L}$

Cross multiply to solve the equation:

$9 \times vol\ in\ L = 6.38$

$vol\ in\ L = \dfrac{6.38}{9}$

$vol\ in\ L = 0.708\ L$

$vol\ in\ ml = 0.708\ \cancel{L} \times \dfrac{1000\ ml}{\cancel{L}}$

$vol\ in\ ml = \textbf{708 ml}$

★ **Example:** *The electrolyte panel on a dog indicates that it is hypokalemic and you determine it needs 4 mEq of potassium chloride (KCl). You have potassium chloride in the pharmacy. The label reads "contains 20 mEq in 10 ml." How many ml of this solution should the dog receive?*

$\dfrac{number\ of\ ml\ required}{dose\ required\ in\ mEq} = \dfrac{ml\ of\ drug\ in\ solution}{mEq\ of\ drug\ in\ solution}$

$$\frac{\text{ml required}}{4 \text{ mEq}} = \frac{10 \text{ ml}}{20 \text{ mEq}}$$

ml required × 20 mEq = 10 ml × 4 mEq

ml required × 20 mEq = 40 mEq/ml

$$\text{ml required} = \frac{40 \text{ mEq} / \text{ml}}{20 \text{ mEq}}$$

ml required = **2 ml**

★ **Example:** *Calcium chloride (CaCl₂) is available as a 1g /10 ml solution, a) what is the concentration of CaCl₂ in milligrams per milliliter? and b) how many mEq of calcium (Ca²⁺) are there in each milliliter of this solution?*

a) To convert g/100 ml to mg/ml first convert the numerator from grams to milligrams:

$$\frac{1 \text{ g}}{10 \text{ ml}} \times \frac{1000 \text{ mg}}{1 \text{ g}} = \frac{1000 \text{ mg}}{10 \text{ ml}}$$

Then reduce the equation:

$$\frac{1000 \text{ mg}}{10 \text{ ml}} = \frac{100 \text{ mg}}{1 \text{ ml}}$$

Alternately this can be accomplished in a single equation:

$$\frac{1 \text{ g}}{10 \text{ ml}} \times \frac{1000 \text{ mg}}{1 \text{ g}} = \frac{1000 \text{ mg}}{10 \text{ ml}} = 100 \text{ mg} / \text{ml}$$

b) For calcium chloride, USP has the chemical structure ($CaCl_2 \cdot 2H_2O$). To calculate the number of milliequivalents in each ml use the equation:

$$\frac{\text{mEq}}{\text{ml}} = \frac{\text{g} / \text{ml}}{\text{mw}} \times \frac{1000 \text{ mg}}{\text{g}} \times \text{valence}$$

Substitute the concentration of the solution:

$$\frac{1 \text{ g}}{100 \text{ ml}} = 0.01 \text{ g} / \text{ml}:$$

$$\text{mEq} / \text{ml} = \frac{0.1 \text{ g} / \text{ml}}{1 \text{ mw}} \times 1000 \times \text{valence}$$

To determine the valence of the ions consider the equation:

$$CaCl_2 = Ca^{2+} + 2 \; Cl^- + 2 \times (2H^+ + O^{2-})$$

Calcium carries two positives charges in this equation (2+); thus, the valence is 2 (See Appendix D). Substituting the charge (valence) of 2 into the equation:

$$\text{mEq/ml} = 0.1 \text{ g/ml/mw} \; (CaCl_2 \cdot 2H_2O) \times 1000 \times 2$$

and the molecular weight of $(CaCl_2 \cdot 2H_2O)$ (See Appendix D):

$$CaCl_2 = Ca^{2+} + 2 \; Cl^-$$
$$Ca = 40.08 \text{ and } Cl = 35.453$$
$$\text{mw } CaCl_2 = 40.08 + (2 \times 35.453)$$
$$\text{mw } CaCl_2 = 40.08 + 70.906$$
$$\text{mw } CaCl_2 = 110.986$$

$$2 \; H_2O = 2 \; (2H^+ + O^{2-})$$
$$H = 1.008 \text{ and } O = 15.996$$
$$\text{mw } 2H_2O = 2 \times [(2 \times 1.008) + 15.996]$$
$$\text{mw } 2H_2O = 2 \times (2.016 + 15.996)$$
$$\text{mw } 2H_2O = 2 \times 18.012$$
$$\text{mw } 2H_2O = 36.024$$

$$\text{mw } (CaCl_2 \cdot 2H_2O) = \text{mw } CaCl_2 + 2 \times \text{mw } H_2O$$
$$\text{mw } CaCl_2 \cdot 2H_2O = 110.986 + (2 \times 18.012)$$
$$\text{mw } CaCl_2 \cdot 2H_2O = 110.986 + 36.024$$
$$\text{mw } CaCl_2 \cdot 2H_2O = 147.01$$

The mEq/ml can then be determined as

$$mEq/ml = \frac{0.1 \cancel{g}/ml}{147} \times \frac{1000 \text{ mg}}{\cancel{g}} \times 2$$

$$mEq/ml = \frac{100 \text{ mg}/ml}{147} \times 2$$

mEq / ml = 0.68 mg / ml × 2

mEq/ml = **1.36**

The label on 10% calcium chloride states that it contains 13.6 mEq/10 ml, which is 1.36 mEq/ml. It also contains 27.3 mg of calcium per ml.

★ **Example:** *If you wish to supplement calcium but have no calcium chloride ($CaCl_2$), how much calcium gluconate (4.8 mEq/10 ml) would you need to provide the same number of mEq as is contained in 10 ml of $CaCl_2$?*

Step 1:
First, determine the number of mEq contained in 10 ml of $CaCl_2$:

required conc (mEq) = conc (mEq/ml) × volume (ml)
required conc (mEq) = 1.36 mEq/ml × 10 ml
required conc (mEq) = 13.6

Step 2:
Next set up a ratio:

$$\frac{mEq \text{ in solution}}{\text{volume of solution}} = \frac{mEq \text{ desired}}{\text{volume required}}$$

$$\frac{4.8 \text{ mEq}}{10 \text{ ml}} = \frac{13.6 \text{ mEq}}{\text{volume ml}}$$

Cross multiple to solve the equation:
Volume needed × 4.8 mEq = 10 ml × 13.6 mEq

$$volume = \frac{13.6 \; \cancel{mEq} \times 10 \; ml}{4.8 \; \cancel{mEq}}$$

volume = **28.3 ml**

★ **Example:** *How many mEq of sodium (Na) are there in a 5 grain sodium bicarbonate (NaHCO₃) tablet?*

$$mEq = \frac{mg}{mw} \times valence$$

Since the milliequivalent equation asks for the weight of the sodium bicarbonate in milligrams, convert from grains to milligrams using the fact that 1 grain = 64.8 mg (See Appendix G):

$$\frac{5 \; \cancel{grains}}{1} \times \frac{64.8 \; mg}{1 \; \cancel{grain}} = 324 \; mg$$

Next the molecular weight should be determined (See Appendix D):

mw $NaHCO_3$ =
(mw Na) + (mw H) + (mw C) + (3 × mw O)
mw $NaHCO_3$ = 22.99 + 1.008 + 12.01 + (3 × 15.999)
mw $NaHCO_3$ = 84

To determine the valence, consider the components of the molecule:

$NaHCO_3 = Na^+ + H_2O + CO_2^-$

The greatest charge (positive or negative) in this equilibrium is 1; therefore, the valence is 1.

These values can now be substituted into the equation:

$$mEq = \frac{mg}{mw} \times valence$$

$$mEq = \frac{324}{84} \times 1$$

mEq = 3.86 mEq NaHCO$_3$/tablet

Alternate Method:
This process could be combined into one step:

$$mEq = \frac{mg}{mw} \times valence$$

$$mEq / tablet = \frac{[5 \text{ grains} \times (64.5 \text{ mg} / 1 \text{ grain})]}{84} \times 1$$

mEq/tablet = **3.84**

★ **Example:** *How many mEq of sodium are contained in 1 L of 0.9% NaCl?*

Step 1:
To use the equation mEq = (mg/mw) × (valence), convert the concentration of NaCl from a percentage to milligrams per liter. The percentage equals the number of grams contained in 100 ml (See Appendix A), thus:

$$0.9\% = \frac{0.9 \text{ g}}{100 \text{ ml}}$$

$$0.9\% = \frac{0.9 \text{ g}}{100 \text{ ml}} \times \frac{1000 \text{ ml}}{1 \text{ L}}$$

0.9 percent = 9.0 g/L

$$\frac{9 \text{ g}}{1 \text{ L}} \times \frac{1000 \text{ mg}}{1 \text{ g}} = \frac{9,000 \text{ mg}}{1 \text{ L}} = 9,000 \text{ mg} / \text{L}$$

Now insert the value in mg/L into the equation:

$$mEq / L = \frac{mg / L}{mw} \times valence$$

$$mEq / L = \frac{9,000}{58.5} \times 1$$

mEq/L = 153.8 ≈ **154**

Practice Problems
(See Appendix H for answers)

49. How much NaCl concentrate (4 mEq/ml) is needed to make 1 liter of 1/2 normal saline (NS) (0.45% NaCl = 77 mEq/L)?

50. How much NaCl concentrate (4 mEq/ml) is needed to make 1 gal of water isotonic (isotonic = 0.9% NaCl)?

51. How much sodium phosphate injection is needed to provide 30 mEq of sodium phosphate if the commercial preparation provides 3 mmoles/ml phosphate and 4 mEq/ml sodium?

52. How many milliliters of KCl injection (2 mEq/ml) is needed to turn 1 L of D5 1/2 NS into D5 1/2 NS with 20 mEq KCl/L?

53. How many milliliters of 10% calcium chloride ($CaCl_2 \cdot 2 \ H_2O$) injection are required to provide 12 mEq of calcium?

Milliosmoles

An osmole is 1 mole of osmotically active particles or 1 mole of solute present in solution. A milliosmole (mOsm) is 1/1000 or 0.001 or 10^{-3} of an osmole. The milliosmole is frequently used as the measurement for osmotic activity in a biological fluid. For comparison purposes, 1 milliosmole of a monovalent ion (eg, Na^+) equals 1 milliequivalent, and 1 milliosmole of a divalent ion (eg, Ca^{2+}) equals 2 milliequivalents.

$$mOsm = mEq \times (\text{number of particles})$$

$$mOsm = \left(\frac{mg}{mw} \times valence\right) \times (\text{number of particles})$$

★ **Example:** *Sodium chloride is available as a 0.9%
solution. How many mOsm of sodium are
there in each ml of this solution?*

$$mOsm = \left(\frac{mg}{mw} \times valence\right) \times (\text{number of particles})$$

To use the equation above, you must first convert the
concentration from a percentage to mg/ml:

By convention, 0.9% = 0.9 g/100 ml

$$0.9\% = \frac{0.9 \, \cancel{g}}{100 \, ml} \times \frac{1000 \, mg}{1 \, \cancel{g}}$$

$$0.9\% = \frac{9 \, mg}{1 \, ml} = 9 \, mg/ml$$

Next determine the molecular weight of sodium
chloride (NaCl) (See Appendix D):

$$NaCl = Na^+ + Cl^-$$
$$mw \, NaCl = mw \, Na + mw \, Cl$$
$$mw \, Na = 22.99 \text{ and } mw \, Cl = 35.45$$
$$mw \, NaCl = 22.99 + 35.34 = 58.33$$

To determine the valence (charge) of sodium chloride,
consider its equation at equilibrium:

$$NaCl = Na^+ + Cl^-$$

At equilibrium, sodium chloride can dissociate into 2 particles and the largest charge (positive or negative) is 1.

To calculate the mOsm/ml of sodium chloride, substitute these values into the equation:

$$mOsm / ml = \left(\frac{mg / ml}{58.33} \times valence \right) \times \# \text{ of particles}$$

$$mOsm / ml = \left[\frac{9 \text{ mg} / ml}{58.33} \times 1 \right] \times 2$$

mOsm / ml = 0.308

Recall that 0.9% sodium chloride is isosmotic with blood (That is, it does not cause hemodilution or hemoconcentration). The osmolarity of blood is approximately 300 mOsm/L; this can be used to check your work by calculating the mOsm/L of 9% sodium chloride:

$$mOsm / L = \frac{mOsm}{ml} \times \frac{1000 \text{ ml}}{1 \text{ L}}$$

$$mOsm / L = \frac{0.308 \text{ mOsm}}{1 \text{ ml}} \times \frac{1000 \text{ ml}}{1 \text{ L}}$$

mOsm / L = 308

You could also calculate mOsm/L using the fact that 0.9% NaCl contains 154 mEq/L.

mOsm = mEq × # of particles

$$mOsm / L = \frac{mEq}{1 \text{ L}} \times \# \text{ of particles}$$

sodium chloride is made up of two particles:

$NaCl = Na + Cl$

$$mOsm / L = \frac{154 \ mEq}{1 \ L} \times 2$$

$mOsm/L = 308$

Practice Problems
(See Appendix H for answers)

54. Determine the number of mOsm/L of 0.45% NaCl.
55. What is the osmolarity of a 3% NaCl solution?
56. Determine the osmolarity of a 1.3% sodium bicarbonate solution.
57. If KCl solution is 2 mEq/ml, what is the mOsm/L?
58. If calcium chloride dihydrate ($CaCl_2 \bullet 2H_2O$) is available as a 10% solution, what is the mOsm/L? (1 Ca + 2 Cl = 3 particles)

Molarity

Molarity (M) is a common method of expressing the concentration of solutions. Molarity is defined as the number of moles of solute per liter of solution.

$$M = \frac{\# \ of \ mole \ solute}{L \ solution} = \frac{\# \ of \ mmoles \ solute}{ml \ solution}$$

A 1 M NaCl (table salt) solution contains 1 mole of NaCl per liter. A 2 M NaCl solution contains 2 moles of NaCl per liter.

★ **Example:** *The molarity of a solution containing 6.42 g of HCl in 2 L can be solved using the equation:*

$$M = \frac{\# \ of \ mole \ solute}{L \ solution} \quad or \quad \frac{\# \ of \ mmoles \ solute}{ml \ solution}$$

However, common units must first be established. The HCl must be converted from grams / liter to moles / L. This can be done using the equation

moles = grams / molecular weight

To use this equation, the molecular weight (mw) of HCl must first be calculated (See Appendix D):

mw HCl = mw H + mw Cl
mw HCl = 1 + 35.45 = 36.45

The equation can then be modified to reflect moles / L:

$$\text{moles / L} = \frac{\text{grams / L}}{\text{mw}}$$

$$M = \frac{6.42 \text{ g / 2 L}}{36.45}$$

M = 0.088

★ **Example:** *How many grams of HCl must be added to 3 L of water to make 3 L of a 1.5 M HCl solution?*

$$M = \frac{\text{moles solute}}{\text{L solution}} = \frac{\text{g / mw}}{\text{L}}$$

The molecular weight (mw) of HCl has previously been calculated as 36.45:

mw HCl = mw H + mw Cl = 1 + 35.45 = 36.45.

Substituting this value into the equation, we can solve for grams of HCl:

$$M = \frac{\text{moles solute}}{\text{L solution}} = \frac{\text{g / mw}}{\text{L}}$$

$$1.5 \text{ M} = \frac{\text{g/L}}{36.45}$$

g / L = 1.5 × 36.45

g / L = 54.675

Since the problem was to determine the number of grams of HCl to be added to 3 L of water to make a 1.5 M solution, we need only to multiply this result by 3 or set up a simple ratio:

$$\frac{54.7 \text{ g}}{1 \text{ L}} = \frac{\text{g HCl}}{3 \text{ L}}$$

Cross multiply to solve the equation:

g HCl = 54.7 × 3

g HCl = **164**

★ **Example:** *To determine the volume of 12 M sulfuric acid needed to prepare 2 L of a 2.5 molar solution, use a ratio as illustrated above or the following equation:*

concentration × volume = concentration × volume

12 M × unknown volume = 2.5 M × 2 L

$$\text{unknown volume} = \frac{2 \text{ L} \times 2.5 \, \cancel{M}}{12 \, \cancel{M}}$$

unknown volume = **0.417 L**

Add 0.417 L of 12 M sulfuric acid to water to make 2 L of 2.5 M sulfuric acid. *Remember, always add acid to water, never add water to acid!*

Practice Problems
(See Appendix H for answers)

59. Determine the molarity of a solution of sodium chloride containing 90 mg/ml.

60. Determine the molarity of a solution that contains 1.2 g of potassium chloride per liter.
61. Determine the molarity of a 23.4% solution of NaCl.
62. Determine the molarity of a solution that contains 1 mg/ml of zinc.
63. Determine the molarity of a solution that contains 0.4 mg/ml of copper. (Assume a valence of 2.)

Normality

Normality (N) of a solution is the number of gram equivalent weights of solute per liter of solution, or the number of milliequivalents of solute per milliliter. It is simply defined as the molarity times the valence.

$$N = \frac{\# \text{ of grams equivalent solute}}{L} = \frac{\# \text{ mEq solute}}{ml}$$

1 N solution of HCl contains 1 mEq of solute per milliliter. 2 N HCl contains 2 mEq HCl per milliliter.

★ **Example:** *Determine the normality of 1.5 M HCl.*

From the definition of molarity recall that:

$$M = \frac{\# \text{ of mole solute}}{L \text{ solution}} = \frac{g / mw}{L}$$

The molecular weight (mw) of HCl had been previously calculated as 36.45:

mw HCl = mw H + mw Cl = 1 + 35.45 = 36.45

Substituting this value into the equation, we can solve for the number of grams of HCl found in a 1.5 M solution:

$$M = \frac{solute}{L \text{ solution}} = \frac{g / mw}{L}$$

$$1.5 \, M = \frac{g}{36.45}$$

$$g = 36.45 \times 1.5$$

$$g = 54.675 \, g \approx 54.7 \, g$$

Place these values in the normality equation to determine the normality of a 1.5 M HCl solution:

$$N = \frac{\# \text{ of mEq solute}}{ml} = \frac{(g / mw) \times valence}{ml}$$

$$N = \frac{54.7}{36.45} \times 1$$

$$N = 1.52$$

Thus, normality is equal to molarity × valence:

$$M = \frac{mg / mw \text{ solute}}{ml}$$

$$N = \frac{\# \text{ of mEq solute}}{ml} = \frac{mg/mw \text{ solute}}{ml} \times valence$$

Practice Problems
(See Appendix H for answers)

64. Determine the normality of 12 M HCl solution.
65. Determine the volume of 12 M HCl required to prepare 1 L of 1 N HCl.
66. Determine the normality of calcium gluconate solution that contains 0.465 mEq/ml.
67. Determine the normality of a solution that contains 1 mg/ml of zinc.
68. Determine the normality of a 0.9% NaCl solution.

Drug Dosing by Body Surface Area for Dogs and Cats

Body surface area (BSA) should be used to calculate the dosage of extremely toxic or potent drugs in order to minimize toxicity. The initial step in calculating the drug dose is to determine the patient's body surface area (m^2).

---

drug dose in (mg / m^2) = BSA $(m^2) \times \dfrac{\text{drug dose (mg)}}{m^2}$

$(m^2) = \dfrac{K^* \times (\text{wt in g})^{0.67}}{10,000}$

*K for dogs and cats = 10.1

★ **Example:** *The dose of vincristine is 0.025 mg/kg. What is the equivalent dose in mg/m²?*

1 m^2 = 29.6 kg (See Appendix C)

drug dose $= \dfrac{29.6 \cancel{\text{ kg}}}{1 \text{ m}^2} \times \dfrac{0.025 \text{ mg}}{1 \cancel{\text{ kg}}}$

drug dose $= \dfrac{(29.6)\,(0.025 \text{ mg})}{1 \text{ m}^2}$

drug dose = **0.74 mg/m²**

★ **Example:** *Your formulary lists a vincristine dose of 0.8 mg/m² for treating canine lymphosarcoma. What is the equivalent mg/kg dose?*

drug dose (mg / kg) = BSA $(m^2) \times \dfrac{\text{drug dose (mg)}}{m^2}$

$$\text{drug dose} = \frac{1 \ \cancel{m^2}}{29.6 \ \text{kg}} \times \frac{0.8 \ \text{mg}}{\cancel{m^2}}$$

drug dose = **0.027 mg/kg**

★ **Example:** *If cyclophosphamide is given at a dose of 250 mg/m², what is the appropriate dose for a 10 kg dog?*

Convert the animal's weight in kilograms to meters squared using Appendix C:

10 kg = 0.48 m²

and solve the equation:

$$\text{drug dose (mg / m}^2) = \text{BSA (m}^2) \times \frac{\text{drug dose (mg)}}{m^2}$$

$$\text{drug dose} = \frac{250 \ \text{mg}}{m^2} \times \frac{0.48 \ m^2}{1}$$

drug dose = **120 mg**

Practice Problems
(See Appendix H for answers)

69. What is the dose for a 32 lb dog, if cytarabine is prescribed at 100 mg/m²?
70. What is the dose of methotrexate in a 12 lb cat, if it is prescribed at 2.5 mg/m²?
71. The maximum cumulative dose of doxorubicin in dogs with susceptible neoplasms is 240 mg/m². How many treatments can a 68 lb dog undergo if it is receiving 10 mg/m²/dose?
72. How much vinblastine per dose should a 72 lb dog receive that is being treated for lymphoma at 2 mg/m²?
73. A 6 kg cat is being treated with 10,000 U/m² of Elspar® intraperitoneally once a week. How many units does the cat receive at each dose?

Dropper Calibration

A dropper may be calibrated by counting the drops of a liquid as they fall into a graduated cylinder until a measurable volume is obtained. The volume of the drop can then be calculated in ml or minims. Standard dropper volumes are 10, 15, and 20 drops (gtt) per milliliter.

★ **Example:** *Clients leave your practice with a prescription for 0.5 ml Amoxidrops®, which comes with its own calibrated dropper. The clients call a few days later and say the pet has chewed up the dropper. They have another dropper but there are no marks on it. What should they do?*

Step 1:

For calibration, have the clients draw water into the dropper and count the number of drops it takes to fill a measuring spoon. You can have them use any measuring spoon: 1/4 tsp, 1/2 tsp, 1 tsp, or 1 Tbs. Then divide the number of drops by the spoon's volume in milliliters to determine the droppers volume in drops per milliliter.

Step 2:

In this case, it takes 25 drops to fill 1/2 tsp and you can use the conversion chart in Appendix G to determine that 1/2 tsp is equal to 2.5 ml. Then divide the number of drops by the volume in milliliters:

$$\frac{25 \text{ drops}}{2.5 \text{ ml}} = 10 \text{ drops / ml}$$

Step 3:

To deliver the desired dose of 0.5 ml, use the formula

$$\text{drops} = \frac{\text{dose (ml)}}{1} \times \frac{\text{drops}}{1 \text{ ml}}$$

$$\text{drops} = \frac{0.5 \text{ ml}}{1} \times \frac{10 \text{ drops}}{1 \text{ ml}}$$

$$\text{drops} = 5$$

★ **Example:** *How long will a 5 ml bottle of Cyclosporine® last if the dropper dispenses 10 drops per ml and you instill 1 drop into each eye twice a day?*

Step 1:
Calculate the total number of doses available:

$$\frac{5 \text{ ml}}{1 \text{ bottle}} \times \frac{10 \text{ drops}}{1 \text{ ml}} = 50 \text{ drops / bottle}$$

Step 2:
Determine the number of drops used per day:

$$\frac{\text{drops used}}{1 \text{ day}} = \frac{\text{dose}}{1 \text{ eye}} \times \text{\# of eyes treated} \times \frac{\text{\# of times}}{1 \text{ day}}$$

$$\text{drops used} = \frac{1 \text{ drop}}{1 \text{ eye}} \times 2 \text{ eyes} \times \frac{2 \text{ times}}{\text{day}}$$

$$\text{drops used} = 4 \text{ drops / day}$$

Step 3:
To determine how long each bottle will last, divide the number of drops available by the number of drops used per day:

$$\text{day's supply / bottle} = \frac{\text{drops / bottle}}{\text{drops used / day}}$$

$$\text{day's supply} = \frac{50 \text{ drops}}{4 \text{ drops / day}}$$

day's supply = **12.5 days**

Practice Problems
(See Appendix H for answers)

74. If a dropper delivers 1 ml in 15 drops, how many drops are needed to provide 2.5 ml?

75. If a 5 ml bottle of Timoptic® lasts for 12.5 days and the directions instruct the owner to instill 1 drop into each eye every 12 hours, how many drops are dispensed per milliliter of medication?

76. If Terramycin® is prescribed at 2 drops per day and a 10 ml bottle lasts 50 days, how many drops are in 1 ml?

77. How many drops are needed to give a dose of 3 ml, if the dropper delivers 10 drops per milliliter?

78. How many milliliters are 16 drops, if the dropper is calibrated and found to deliver 20 drops per milliliter?

Density

Density is the quantity of matter in a given space as in

16 / gal or g/cm^3 = g/ml

By convention, the density of water = 1 g/ml. One ml of mercury weighs 13.6 g. Therefore, the density of mercury = 13.6 g/ml while the density of water is 1.

Converting Weights to Volumes
(See Appendix G.)

Dairy producers often express production in pounds produced per day. To convert pounds to gallons: divide the number of pounds by the specific gravity of the fluid times 8.33 (the weight of 1 gallon of water).

$$gallons = \frac{pounds}{specific\ gravity \times 8.33}$$

Background information: Each gallon of water contains 3,785 ml and weighs 3,785 g. Since there are

454 g in 1 lb, 3,785 g × (1 lb/454 g) = 8.33 lb. Therefore, each gallon of water weighs 8.33 lb. By convention, the specific gravity of water is 1.

★ **Example:** *If a Jersey cow produces 30 lb / day, how many gallons of milk is produced each day? The specific gravity of milk is assumed to be equal to water or 1.*

$$\text{\# of gallons} = \frac{\text{\# of pounds}}{\text{specific gravity} \times 8.33}$$

$$\text{gallons} = \frac{30 \text{ lb / day}}{1 \times 8.33 \text{ lb}}$$

gallons = **3.6 gallons**

★ **Example:** *If a Holstein cow produces 6 gallons per day, how many pounds of milk per day does she produce?*

$$\frac{\text{\# of gallons}}{\text{day}} = \frac{\text{\# of pounds}}{\text{specific gravity} \times 8.33}$$

$$\frac{6 \text{ gallons}}{\text{day}} = \frac{\text{pounds / day}}{1 \times 8.33}$$

Cross multiply to solve the equation:

pounds = 6 × 8.33

pounds = **50 lb**

★ **Example:** *You have a 55 gallon drum that is partially filled with a malathion parasiticide that you want to apply to a group of cattle. You know that the liquid in the barrel weighs 260 lb. How many gallons of parasiticide are in the drum (assuming a specific gravity of 1)?*

$$\text{\# of gallons} = \frac{\text{\# of pounds}}{\text{specific gravity} \times 8.33}$$

$$\text{gallons} = \frac{260 \text{ lb}}{1 \times 8.33}$$

gallons = **31.2 gal**

Practice Problems
(See Appendix H for answers)

79. How many pounds of milk per day does a Brown Swiss produce if its average production is 4.2 gallons per day?
80. If a Charlais calf is drinking 2.5 gallons per day, how many pounds of milk is it drinking?
81. If a substance has a specific gravity of 0.8, how many pounds are contained in 1 gallon of this substance?
82. How much does 2 gal of a substance weigh that has a specific gravity of 1.2?
83. What is the specific gravity of a substance if 7 gallons weigh 34 lb?

Math Basics
Part 2

Dilutions

Dilutions are useful when very small quantities of a drug or solution are required. Dilutions are commonly used when the amount of drug or solution to be given is so small that it cannot be accurately measured or the drug's formulation does not allow for the accurate or easy administration of the prescribed dose.

★ **Example:** *What volume of ivermectin will be required to treat a 30 g parakeet for mites using a dose of 200 mcg/kg of ivermectin? The commercially available ivermectin preparation is a 1% solution.*

Step 1:
First, convert the parakeet's weight from grams to kilograms (See Appendix G):

$$\text{wt in kg} = \frac{\text{wt (g)}}{1} \times \frac{1 \text{ kg}}{1000 \text{ g}}$$

$$\text{wt in kg} = \frac{30 \text{ g}}{1} \times \frac{1 \text{ kg}}{1000 \text{ g}} = \frac{30}{1000} = 0.03 \text{ kg}$$

Step 2:
Determine the dose required in micrograms:

$$\text{dose (mcg)} = \frac{\text{dose in mcg}}{1 \text{ kg}} \times \frac{\text{wt (kg)}}{1}$$

$$\text{dose (mcg)} = \frac{200}{1 \text{ kg}} \times \frac{0.03 \text{ kg}}{1}$$

$$\text{dose} = (200 \text{ mcg}) \times (0.03 \text{ kg}) = 6 \text{ mcg}$$

Step 3:
If the commercial preparation is 1%, how much is needed for each dose? Convert the concentration from percentage to mcg/ml (See Appendix G):

$$\% = \frac{g}{100 \text{ ml}}$$

$$1 \% = \frac{1 \text{ g}}{100 \text{ ml}}$$

$$1 \% = \frac{1 \cancel{g}}{100 \text{ ml}} \times \frac{1000 \text{ mg}}{1 \cancel{g}}$$

$$1 \% = \frac{1000 \text{ mg}}{100 \text{ ml}}$$

$$1 \% = \frac{10 \text{ mg}}{1 \text{ ml}}$$

$$\text{dose} = \frac{10 \cancel{mg}}{1 \text{ ml}} \times \frac{1000 \text{ mcg}}{1 \cancel{mg}}$$

dose = 10,000 mcg/ml

Step 4:
To determine the volume required for the parakeet's 6 mcg dose, set up a ratio:

$$\frac{6 \text{ mcg}}{10,000 \text{ mcg}} = \frac{\text{volume needed in ml}}{1 \text{ ml}}$$

Cross multiply to solve the equation.

volume required in ml × 10,000 = 6

$$\text{volume required} = \frac{6 \cancel{mcg}}{10,000 \cancel{mcg}}$$

volume required = 0.0006 ml

Alternate Step 4:
Use the equation:
concentration × volume = concentration × volume

10,000 × volume needed in ml = 6 mcg × 1 ml

volume needed in ml $= \dfrac{6 \text{ mcg} \times 1 \text{ ml}}{10,000 \text{ mcg}} = 0.0006$ ml

Step 5:
Since 0.0006 ml could not be accurately measured, a dilution should be made. A 1:100 dilution can be made by mixing 1 part ivermectin with 99 parts propylene glycol. This can be made by adding 0.1 ml of ivermectin to 9.9 ml of propylene glycol or 1 ml of ivermectin to 99 ml propylene glycol if you have a whole aviary to treat.

Step 6:
Assume you have an aviary to treat and have diluted 1 ml ivermectin with 99 ml of propylene glycol. You now have 100 ml of solution that contains 10,000 mcg of ivermectin. What volume is needed for the 6 mcg dose? (See Appendix G)

Working solution $= \dfrac{10,000 \text{ mcg}}{100 \text{ ml}}$ or $\dfrac{100 \text{ mcg}}{1 \text{ ml}}$

Set up a ratio to determine the volume of the diluted solution required to obtain a 6 mcg dose:

$\dfrac{6 \text{ mcg}}{100 \text{ mcg}} = \dfrac{\text{required volume ml}}{1 \text{ ml}}$

Cross multiply to solve the equation:

required volume × 100 = 6 × 1

$$\text{required volume} = \frac{6 \cancel{\text{mcg}}}{100 \cancel{\text{mcg}}}$$

required volume = 0.06 ml

★ **Example:** *If a flock of 100 cockatiels is to receive 40 mg/kg q24h of ciprofloxacin in the drinking water and each cockatiel weighs approximately 90 g, how much ciprofloxacin is needed per day?*

As in the previous example, the weight of the birds must be converted from grams to kilograms. Then multiply the dose in milligrams per kilograms per day by the weight of each animal in kilograms. Finally, this dose must be multiplied by the number of birds (100) that are to receive it.

Step 1:
Convert the cockatiel's weight from grams to kilograms (See Appendix G):

$$\text{wt in kg} = \text{wt (g)} \times \frac{1 \text{ kg}}{1000 \text{ g}}$$

$$\text{wt in kg} = \frac{90 \cancel{g}}{1} \times \frac{1 \text{ kg}}{1000 \cancel{g}}$$

$$\text{wt in kg} = \frac{90}{1000} = 0.09 \text{ kg}$$

Step 2:
b) Determine dose required in mg/day:

$$\text{dose in mg} = \frac{\text{dose (mg)}}{1 \text{ kg}} \times \frac{\text{wt (kg)}}{1}$$

$$\text{dose in mg} = \frac{40 \text{ mg / day}}{1 \cancel{\text{kg}}} \times \frac{0.09 \cancel{\text{kg}}}{1} = 3.6 \text{ mg / day}$$

Step 3:
Multiply the dose in milligrams by the number of cockatiels that are to receive it:

$$\frac{3.6 \text{ mg}}{1 \text{ day}} \times \frac{100 \text{ birds}}{1} = 360 \text{ mg / day}$$

Alternate Steps 1 to 3:
Steps (1) through (3) can be combined into a single calculation:

$$\text{dose / day} = \frac{\text{birds} \times \text{bird's wt (g)}}{1} \times \frac{1 \text{ kg}}{1000 \text{ g}} \times \frac{\text{dose (mg/day)}}{1 \text{ kg}}$$

$$\text{dose / day} = \frac{100 \text{ birds} \times 90 \text{ g/bird}}{1} \times \frac{1 \text{ kg}}{1000 \text{ g}} \times \frac{40 \text{ mg/day}}{1 \text{ kg}}$$

$$\text{dose/day} = \frac{100 \times 90 \times 40 \text{ mg / day}}{1000}$$

dose / day = 360 mg/day

Step 4:
Ciprofloxacin is available as a 500 mg tablet. To determine the number of tablets needed to treat the flock for 7 days, multiply the dose per day by 7 days and then divide the result by 500 mg:

$$\text{total dose} = \frac{\text{dose}}{\text{day}} \times 7 \text{ days}$$

$$\text{total dose} = \frac{360 \text{ mg}}{1 \text{ day}} \times \frac{7 \text{ days}}{1} = 2520 \text{ mg}$$

$$\text{tablets needed} = \frac{2520 \text{ mg}}{500 \text{ mg / tablet}} = 5.04 \text{ tablets}$$

★ **Example:** *You send clients home with directions to dilute chlorhexidine 1:40 to soak their animal's foot for 10 minutes once a day. Use household measurements of teaspoons (5 ml) and cups (240 ml) to make this 1:40 solution.*

Step 1:

Set a ratio to determine how much chlorhexidine should be added to each cup of water:

Remember to add 1 to 40 for the total solution volume.

$$\frac{1}{41} = \frac{\text{volume needed in ml}}{1 \text{ cup}}$$

$$\frac{1}{41} = \frac{\text{volume needed in ml}}{240 \text{ ml}}$$

volume needed × 41 = 240 × 1

$$\text{volume needed} = \frac{240}{41}$$

volume needed ≈ 5.85 ml

Step 2:

Next convert from milliliters to teaspoons using the fact that 1 tsp = 5 ml (See Appendix G):

$$\frac{5.85 \text{ ml}}{1} \times \frac{1 \text{ tsp}}{5 \text{ ml}} = 1.17 \text{ tsp}$$

Thus, a 1:40 solution ≈ **1 1/4 tsp in 1 cup of warm water**

★ **Example:** *A 0.05% solution of chlorhexidine is suggested to irrigate tissues during surgery. How much of a commercial 2% solution should be added to 1 L of H_2O for irrigation?*

Step 1:
concentration × volume = concentration × volume

0.05% × 1 L = 2% × required volume (L)

$$\text{required volume} = \frac{0.05 \times 1 \text{ L}}{2}$$

required volume = 0.025 L

Step 2:
Convert from liters to milliliters using the fact that
1 L = 1000 ml (See Appendix G):

$$\frac{0.025 \cancel{\text{ L}}}{1} \times \frac{1000 \text{ ml}}{1 \cancel{\text{ L}}} = 25 \text{ ml}$$

Thus, add **25 ml** of a 2% solution to each liter of water
to make a 0.05% solution.

★ **Example:** *If Betadine®, a 10% povidone-iodine
solution, is diluted 1:213, what percentage is
the resulting solution?*

Step 1:
Set up a ratio with like units in both the numerator
and the denominator:

Remember to add 1 to 213 for the total solution.

$$\frac{1}{214} = \frac{\% \text{ unknown solution}}{10 \text{ \%}}$$

Cross multiply to solve the equation:

% of unknown × 214 = 10 × 1

$$\% \text{ of unknown} = \frac{10 \times 1}{214}$$

% of unknown ≈ 0.0467% ≈ 0.05%

Step 2:

How many parts per million (ppm) would the resulting 0.05% solution be? For this calculation, first convert 0.05% to g/ml: (See Appendix G)

$$\% = \frac{g}{100 \text{ ml}}$$

Thus,

$$0.05\% = \frac{0.05 \text{ g}}{100 \text{ ml}}$$

Next, set up the ratio of parts per million is equal to grams per 1,000,000 milliliters (See Appendix G):

ppm = g/1,000,000ml

$$\frac{0.05 \text{ g}}{100 \text{ ml}} = \frac{\text{unknown g}}{1,000,000 \text{ ml}}$$

unknown × 100 ml = 0.05 × 1,000,000 ml

$$\text{unknown} = \frac{0.05 \times 1,000,000 \text{ ml}}{100 \text{ ml}}$$

$$\text{unknown} = \frac{50,000}{100}$$

unknown = **500 ppm**

★ **Example:** *Sodium bicarbonate ($NaHCO_3$) is commercially available as a 7.5% solution. If a 1.3% solution is isotonic, how much of the 7.5% solution should be added to a 250 ml bag of water to make the final solution isotonic?*

Step 1:

concentration × volume = concentration × volume

7.5% × required ml = 1.3% × 250 ml

$$\text{required ml} = \frac{0.013 \times 250}{0.075}$$

required ml = 43.3 ml

Step 2:

Withdraw 43.3 ml of water and then add 43.3 ml of the 7.5% sodium bicarbonate solution to the 206.7 ml of water (250 ml – 43.3 ml) to make a 1.3% solution.

Alternate Method:

The amount of 7.5% sodium bicarbonate that should be added directly to 250 ml of water can be determined by using the equation:

7.5% × required ml = 1.3% × (250 + required ml)

0.075 × required ml = 0.013 × (250 + required ml)

0.075 × required ml = 0.013 × (required ml) + 0.013 × (250)

Move the unknown to the same side by subtracting from each side of the equation.

0.075 × (required ml) – 0.013 × (required ml) = 3.25 ml

0.062 × (required ml) = 3.25 ml

$$\text{required ml} = \frac{3.25 \text{ ml}}{0.062}$$

required ml = **52.4 ml**

Add 52.4 ml of the 7.5% solution to 250 ml.

★ **Example:** *What volume of a 5% sodium bicarbonate solution would be required to make 250 ml of water isotonic?*

concentration × volume = concentration × volume

5% × required ml = 1.3% × 250 ml

Convert percentages to decimal:

0.05 × required ml = 0.013 × 250 ml

$$required\ ml = \frac{0.013 \times 250\ ml}{0.05}$$

required ml = 65 ml

Withdraw and discard 65 ml of sterile water from the bag and add 65 ml of 5% sodium bicarbonate solution. Since 5% is less concentrated than 7.5%, it makes sense that it would take more 5% solution to make the same volume isotonic.

★ **Example:** *Using the dry powder, how much sodium bicarbonate would be required to make 250 ml of water isotonic (1.3% solution)? Assume the powdered sodium bicarbonate ($NaHCO_3$) to be of analytical quality and almost entirely free of impurities (100% $NaHCO_3$):*

Convert the 1.3% to grams (g) per 100 ml:

$$\% = \frac{g}{100\ ml}$$

$$1.3\% = \frac{1.3\ g}{100\ ml}$$

$$\frac{1.3\ g}{required\ g} = \frac{100\ ml}{250\ ml}$$

Cross multiply to solve the equation:

required g × 100 ml = 250 ml × 1.3 g

$$\text{required g} = \frac{250 \text{ ml} \times 1.3 \text{ g}}{100 \text{ ml}}$$

required g = **3.25 g**

Practice Problems
(See Appendix H for answers)

84. How much aminophylline 25 mg/ml solution is required to make 1 L of 1 mg/ml?

85. How much potassium acetate injection (2 mEq/ml) is required to fill an order of 3 L of D_5 1/2 NS with 40 mEq/L potassium acetate?

86. If 1 ampule (10 ml) of 10% calcium gluconate contains 0.465 mEq/ml and is added to 100 ml of D_5W, what is the resulting concentration of calcium in mEq/ml?

87. How much absolute alcohol (100%) is needed to make 1 L of 10% alcohol to treat antifreeze toxicity?

88. How many gallons of 0.5% sodium hypochlorite can be made from 1 gal of the 5% commercial preparation?

Drug Dosing

The calculation of the quantity of drug to administer is commonly based on the patient's weight, or in the case of more potentially toxic drugs—body surface area (BSA). Drug dosing may also require converting units of measure.

Converting Micrograms to Milliliters

★ **Example:** *DDAVP is prescribed to treat von Willebrandt's disease in dogs at 1 mcg/kg. The commercial preparation is a 0.01% solution. How much DDAVP is needed to treat a 70 lb dog?*

Step 1:
Convert the weight of the dog from pounds to kilograms:

$$\frac{70 \text{ lb}}{1} \times \frac{1 \text{ kg}}{2.2 \text{ lb}} = 31.8 \text{ kg}$$

Step 2:
Multiply the weight in kilograms by the dose of 1 mcg/kg:

$$\frac{31.8 \text{ kg}}{1} \times \frac{1 \text{ mcg}}{\text{kg}} = 31.8 \text{ mcg}$$

Step 3:
Convert to common units and divide the dose by the strength of the commercial solution to determine the number of milliliters required:

$$\% = \frac{\text{g}}{100 \text{ ml}}$$

$$0.01\% = \frac{0.01 \text{ g}}{100 \text{ ml}}$$

By definition:

1 g = 1000 mg and 1 mg = 1000 mcg
(See Appendix G)

$$0.01\% = \frac{0.01 \text{ g}}{100 \text{ ml}} \times \frac{1000 \text{ mg}}{1 \text{ g}} \times \frac{1000 \text{ mcg}}{\text{mg}}$$

0.01% = 100 mcg/ml

$$\text{required dose} = \frac{31.8 \text{ mcg}}{0.01\%}$$

$$\text{required dose} = \frac{\dfrac{31.8 \text{ mcg}}{100 \text{ mcg}}}{\text{ml}}$$

$$\text{required dose} = \frac{\dfrac{31.8 \text{ mcg}}{1}}{\dfrac{100 \text{ mcg}}{\text{ml}}}$$

Step 4:

$$\text{required dose} = \frac{31.8 \text{ \sout{mcg}}}{1} \times \frac{1 \text{ ml}}{100 \text{ \sout{mcg}}}$$

required dose = 0.318 ml ≈ **0.32 ml**

Converting Dose in Milligrams to Number of Tablets

★ **Example:** *Trimethoprim-sulfa (TMS) is available in 30 mg, 120 mg, 480 mg, and 960 mg tablets. The largest size tablets (960 mg) contain 800 mg sulfa and 160 trimethoprim (TM). How many tablets are needed to treat a 1000 lb horse at 4 mg/kg, based on the trimethoprim, orally every 12 hours for 10 days?*

Step 1:
Convert the weight of the horse from pounds to kilograms (See Appendix G):

$$\frac{1000 \text{ \sout{lb}}}{1} \times \frac{1 \text{ kg}}{2.2 \text{ \sout{lb}}} = 454 \text{ kg}$$

Step 2:
How many tablets are needed per dose?

$$\frac{454 \text{ \sout{kg}}}{1} \times \frac{4 \text{ mg TM / dose}}{1 \text{ \sout{kg}}} = 1{,}816 \text{ mg TM / dose}$$

$$\frac{1{,}816 \text{ \sout{mg TM} / dose}}{160 \text{ \sout{mg TM} / tablet}} = 11.35 \text{ tablets / dose}$$

Round this dose off to 11.5 tablets per dose because the tablets are scored in half but cannot accurately be broken into thirds.

Step 3:
Calculate the number of tablets needed to treat this horse for 10 days:

$$\text{tablets needed} = \frac{\text{\# of tablets}}{1 \text{ dose}} \times \frac{\text{\# of doses}}{\text{day}} \times \text{\# of days of tx}$$

$$\text{tablets needed} = \frac{11.5 \text{ tablets}}{1 \text{ dose}} \times \frac{2 \text{ doses}}{1 \text{ day}} \times 10 \text{ days}$$

tablets needed = **230 tablets**

Converting the Dose in Milligrams to Milliliters of an Injectable Product

★ **Example:** *A fox kit needs trimethoprim-sulfa (TMS) at 10 mg/lb subcutaneously every 12 hours for 14 days. If the kit weighs 2.5 kg, how much TMS is needed a) per dose, and b) for 14 days of treatment?*

Convert the weight of the animal from kilograms to pounds (See Appendix G):

wt (kg) × (2.2 lb/kg) = wt (lb)

$$\frac{2.5 \text{ kg}}{1} \times \frac{2.2 \text{ lb}}{1 \text{ kg}} = 5.5 \text{ lb}$$

a) To determine the amount of TMS required per dose, multiply the dose by the weight of the animal:

$$\frac{5.5 \text{ lb}}{1} \times \frac{10 \text{ mg dose}}{\text{lb}} = 55 \text{ mg / dose}$$

Tribrissen® is available as a 24% and 48% injection.

Calculate the volume of the 24% solution required per dose:

$$\% = \frac{g}{100 \text{ ml}}$$

$$24\% = \frac{24 \text{ g}}{100 \text{ ml}}$$

$$24\% = \frac{24 \text{ g}}{100 \text{ ml}} \times \frac{1000 \text{ mg}}{1 \text{ g}}$$

$$24\% = 240 \text{ mg/ml}$$

$$\text{volume required} = \frac{\text{dose (mg)}}{\text{concentration (mg / ml)}}$$

$$\text{volume required} = \frac{55 \text{ mg}}{240 \text{ mg} / \text{ml}}$$

$$\text{volume required} = 0.23 \text{ ml}$$

b) To determine the amount of TMS needed for 14 days of therapy, multiply the milligrams/dose required by the number of doses required per day by the number of days of therapy:

$$\text{total mg required} = \frac{\text{mg/dose}}{1} \times \frac{\text{\# of doses}}{1 \text{ day}} \times \text{days of therapy}$$

$$\text{total mg required} = \frac{55 \text{ mg / dose}}{1} \times \frac{2 \text{ doses}}{1 \text{ day}} \times 14 \text{ days}$$

$$\text{total mg required} = 1,540 \text{ mg}$$

Calculate the volume of the 24% solution required to complete the therapy:

$$\% = \frac{g}{100 \text{ ml}}$$

$$24\% = \frac{24 \text{ g}}{100 \text{ ml}}$$

$$24\% = \frac{24 \text{ g}}{100 \text{ ml}} \times \frac{1000 \text{ mg}}{1 \text{ g}}$$

24% = 240 mg/ml

volume required =

$$\frac{\text{dose (mg)}}{\text{conc (mg / ml)}} \times \frac{\text{\# of doses}}{1 \text{ day}} \times \text{\# of days of therapy}$$

$$\text{volume required} = \frac{55 \cancel{\text{mg}}}{240 \cancel{\text{mg}}/\text{ml}} \times \frac{2 \cancel{\text{doses}}}{1 \cancel{\text{dose/day}}} \times 14 \cancel{\text{days}}$$

$$\text{volume required} = \frac{55 \times 2 \times 14}{240} \text{ ml}$$

$$\text{volume required} = \frac{1540}{240} \text{ ml}$$

volume required = **6.4 ml**

Practice Problems
(See Appendix H for answers)

89. DDAVP is now available in tablet form. The 0.2 mg tablet is equivalent to 10 mcg of the intranasal preparation. The 0.4 mg tablet is equivalent to 20 mcg of the intranasal preparation. If diabetes

insipidus was previously treated with 0.1 ml of the 0.01% preparation, what is the oral equivalent dose?

90. How many milliliters of 48% Tribrissen® are needed to treat a 30 kg dog for 7 days, if the recommended dose is 10 mg/lb every 12 hours?

91. Calcium gluconate is 6.5% calcium by weight. How much calcium gluconate is need to provide 115 mg of calcium?

92. How much calcium gluconate is needed to provide 90 mg of calcium, if calcium gluconate is 9% calcium by weight?

93. How much calcium carbonate is contained in one Os-Cal 500®? (Calcium carbonate is 40% calcium by weight. Os-Cal 500® contains 500 mg of calcium).

Emergency Drugs

Converting Ratios, Percentages, and Milligrams per Milliliter

★ **Example:** *Epinephrine is available as a 1:10,000 preparation. What is the a) mg/ml concentration and b) concentration percentage?*

a) To determine the mg/ml concentration:

By definition, $1:10,000 = \dfrac{1 \text{ g}}{10,000 \text{ ml}}$

Convert grams to milligrams:

$$1:10,000 = \frac{1 \, \cancel{g}}{10,000 \text{ ml}} \times \frac{1000 \text{ mg}}{1 \, \cancel{g}}$$

$$1:10,000 = \frac{1000 \text{ mg}}{10,000 \text{ ml}}$$

$$1{:}10{,}000 = \frac{1 \text{ mg}}{10 \text{ ml}}$$

1:10,000 = **0.1 mg/ml**

b) To determine the concentration percentage:

$$\% = \frac{g}{100 \text{ ml}}$$

$$1{:}10{,}000 = \frac{1 \text{ g}}{10{,}000 \text{ mg}}$$

$$\% = \frac{1 \text{ g}}{10{,}000 \text{ ml}} \times \frac{100 \text{ ml}}{1 \text{ g}}$$

$$\% = \frac{100}{10{,}000}$$

$$\% = \frac{1}{100}$$

% = **0.01%**

★ **Example:** *What is the mg/ml concentration of 1% atropine? Express the percentage as a ratio.*

$$1\% = \frac{1 \text{ g}}{100 \text{ ml}} = \frac{1000 \text{ mg}}{100 \text{ g}} = \frac{1000 \text{ mg}}{10{,}000 \text{ ml}} = 10 \text{ mg} / \text{ml}$$

Express this percentage as a ratio:

$$1\% = \frac{1 \text{ g}}{100 \text{ ml}} = 1{:}100$$

★ **Example:** *Lidocaine 2% is used as an intravenous drip at 2 mg/min. How much 2% lidocaine should be added to 500 ml of fluid to make a concentration of 2 mg/ml?*

Step 1:

$$\% = \frac{g}{100 \text{ ml}}$$

Therefore, $2\% = \dfrac{2 \text{ g}}{100 \text{ ml}}$

Convert grams to milligrams (See Appendix G):

$$\frac{2 \cancel{\text{g}}}{100 \text{ ml}} \times \frac{1000 \text{ mg}}{1 \cancel{\text{g}}} = \frac{2000 \text{ mg}}{100 \text{ ml}} = 20 \text{ mg / ml}$$

Step 2:

concentration × volume = concentration × volume

(20 mg/ml) × unknown volume = 2 mg/ml × 500 ml

20 mg/ml × unknown volume = 1000 mg

$$\text{unknown volume} = \frac{1000 \cancel{\text{mg}}}{20 \cancel{\text{mg}} / \text{ml}}$$

unknown volume = 50 ml

Step 3:

Add 50 ml of 2% lidocaine to 500 ml to make a 2 mg/ml solution.

★ **Example:** *200 mg of dopamine in 500 ml of fluids is what a) mg/ml, b) mcg/ml, c) percentage, and d) ratio?*

a) To determine mg / ml:

$$\frac{200 \text{ mg}}{500 \text{ ml}} = 0.4 \text{ mg/ml}$$

b) To determine mcg / ml, see Appendix G:

$$\frac{0.4 \text{ mg}}{1 \text{ ml}} \times \frac{1000 \text{ mcg}}{1 \text{ mg}} = 400 \text{ mcg/ml}$$

c) To determine the percentage, first:
Convert milligrams to grams:

$$\frac{200 \text{ mg}}{500 \text{ ml}} \times \frac{1 \text{ g}}{1000 \text{ mg}}$$

$$= \frac{200 \text{ g}}{50,000 \text{ ml}} = 0.004 \text{ g / ml}$$

By definition, % = g / 100 ml

Thus, $\dfrac{0.004 \text{ g}}{\text{ml}} \times \dfrac{\text{unknown g}}{100 \text{ ml}}$

unknown g = 100 × 0.004 g

unknown g = 0.04 g

% = 0.04

d) To determine the ratio:

By definition $0.04\% = \dfrac{0.04 \text{ g}}{100 \text{ ml}}$

$$\text{ratio} = \frac{\text{volume in ml}}{\text{weight in g}}$$

$$\text{ratio} = \frac{100 \text{ ml}}{0.04 \text{ g}}$$

ratio = **1:2,500**

★ **Example:** *Isoproteronol is commercially available as 1 g / 5 ml concentration. What is the final concentration if this solution is in a) mg/ml, b) mcg/ml, c) a percentage concentration, and d) a ratio if 1 g isoproteronol is in 250 ml of D_5W?*

a) To determine mg / ml: Convert grams to milligrams (See Appendix G):

$$\frac{1\ \cancel{g}}{250\ \text{ml}} \times \frac{1000\ \text{mg}}{1\ \cancel{g}}$$

$$\text{concentration} = \frac{1000\ \text{mg}}{250\ \text{ml}}$$

concentration = **4 mg/ml**

b) To determine mcg / ml: Convert milligrams to micrograms (See Appendix G):

$$\frac{4\ \cancel{mg}}{1\ \text{ml}} \times \frac{1000\ \text{mcg}}{1\ \cancel{mg}} = 4{,}000\ \text{mcg / ml}$$

c) To determine the percentage concentration:

$$\frac{1\ \text{g}}{250\ \text{ml}} = \frac{\text{unknown g}}{100\ \text{ml}}$$

Cross multiply to solve the equation:

$$250 \times \text{unknown g} = 100 \times 1$$

$$\text{unknown g} = \frac{100}{250}$$

unknown g = 0.4 g

Thus, % = **0.4**

d) To determine the ratio:

$$\frac{0.4\ \text{g}}{100\ \text{ml}} = 0.4\,\%$$

$$\text{ratio} = \frac{\text{volume in ml}}{\text{weight in g}}$$

$$\text{ratio} = \frac{100 \text{ ml}}{0.4 \text{ g}}$$

ratio = **1:250**

★ **Example:** *Ten milliliters of dobutamine (250 mg/10 ml) is diluted in 240 ml D$_5$W or 0.9% NaCl to make a total volume of 250 ml. Express the resulting solution as a a) ratio, b) percentage, and c) mcg/ml.*

a) To determine the ratio: Convert milligrams to grams (See Appendix G):

$$\frac{250 \text{ mg}}{250 \text{ ml}} \times \frac{0.001 \text{ g}}{1 \text{ mg}} = \frac{0.25 \text{ g}}{250 \text{ ml}}$$

$$\text{ratio} = \frac{\text{volume in ml}}{\text{weight in g}}$$

$$\text{ratio} = \frac{250}{0.25}$$

ratio = **1:1000**

b) To determine the percentage:

$$\frac{0.25 \text{ g}}{250 \text{ ml}} = \frac{\text{unknown g}}{100 \text{ ml}}$$

Cross multiply to solve the equation:

unknown g × 250 ml = 0.25 g × 100 ml

$$\text{unknown g} = \frac{0.25 \text{ g} \times 100 \text{ ml}}{250 \text{ ml}}$$

unknown g = 0.1 g

By convention, $\dfrac{0.1 \text{ g}}{100 \text{ ml}} = 0.1\%$

c) To determine mcg / ml:

$$\frac{250 \text{ mg}}{250 \text{ ml}} = \frac{1 \text{ mg}}{1 \text{ ml}}$$

Convert milligrams to micrograms
(See Appendix G):

$$\frac{1 \text{ mg}}{1 \text{ ml}} \times \frac{1000 \text{ mcg}}{1 \text{ mg}} = 1000 \text{ mcg / ml}$$

I.V. Drips and Solutions

I.V. Drips

concentration in mg/ml = mg of drug/ml of I.V. fluids

For I.V. drips, the flow rate in milliliters per hour can be determined by dividing the number of milliliters to be delivered by the number of hours in which it is to be delivered. The number of milliliters per minute can be determined by dividing the number obtained from this calculation by 60.

$$\text{ml per hour} = \frac{\text{volume to be infused in ml}}{\text{length of infusion in hr}}$$

$$\text{ml per minute} = \frac{\text{volume to be infused in ml}}{\text{length of infusion in hr} \times (60 \text{ min/hour})}$$

$$\text{drip rate} = \frac{\text{ml required}}{\text{time}} \times \frac{\text{drops}}{1 \text{ ml}}$$

When determining the flow rate for I.V. solutions, it is important to note that the number of drops (gtt) of solution/ml will vary with the type of I.V. set. Standard drip sets are calibrated for 10, 15, or 20 drops/ml for aqueous solutions and microdrop sets are calibrated for 60 drops/ml.

★ **Example**: *Convert the infusion of 1 liter per day to milliliters per minute.*

Step 1:

Convert from liters to milliliters (See Appendix G):

$$\frac{1 \, \cancel{L}}{1 \, \text{day}} \times \frac{1000 \, \text{ml}}{1 \, \cancel{L}} = \frac{1000 \, \text{ml}}{1 \, \text{day}}$$

Step 2:
Convert from days to minutes:

$$\frac{1000 \, \text{ml}}{1 \, \cancel{\text{day}}} \times \frac{1 \, \cancel{\text{day}}}{24 \, \cancel{\text{hr}}} \times \frac{1 \, \cancel{\text{hr}}}{60 \, \text{min}} = 0.69 \, \text{ml} / \text{min}$$

Step 3:
Using a specific drip set, the rate can be determined by multiplying the rate in ml/min × gtt/ml. The number of drops per minute may be approximated for each type of drip set. Using a 10 gtt / min set:

$$\frac{0.69 \, \cancel{\text{ml}}}{1 \, \text{min}} \times \frac{10 \, \text{gtt}}{1 \, \cancel{\text{ml}}} \approx 7 \text{gtt} / \text{min}$$

Using a 15 gtt/min set:

$$\frac{0.69 \, \cancel{\text{ml}}}{1 \, \text{min}} \times \frac{15 \, \text{gtt}}{1 \, \cancel{\text{ml}}} \approx 10 \, \text{gtt} / \text{min}$$

A table of approximated flow rates follows using the commonly available administration (adm) sets to deliver 1/2, 1, or 3 L per day.

Adm Set (approx.)*	500ml/day (≈ 21 ml/hr)	1000 ml/day (≈ 42 ml/hr)	3 L/day (≈125 ml/hr)
10 gtt/ml	3.5 gtt/min	7 gtt/min	21 gtt/min
15 gtt/ml	5 gtt/min	10 gtt/min	31 gtt/min
20 gtt/ml	7 gtt/min	14 gtt/min	42 gtt/min
60 gtt/ml	21 gtt/min	42 gtt/min	125 gtt/min

when administering aqueous solutions

I.V. Solutions

$$\text{concentration in mg / ml} = \frac{\text{mg of drug}}{\text{ml of I.V. fluids}}$$

$$\text{drops / minute} = \text{rate} = \left(\frac{\text{ml}}{\text{min}} \times \frac{\text{drops}}{\text{ml}} \right)$$

$$\text{dose (mcg/min)} = \text{dose (mcg/kg/min)} \times \text{wt (kg)}$$

$$\text{volume (ml)} = \frac{\text{dose (mcg / min)}}{\text{concentration (mcg / ml)}}$$

$$\text{rate (ml / min)} = \frac{\text{concentration / hour}}{\text{concentration / ml}}$$

$$\text{medication dose / hr} = \frac{\text{mg of drug} \times \text{flow rate (ml / hr)}}{\text{ml of solution}}$$

★ **Example:** *What is the resulting concentration (in mcg/ml) when 50 mg of sodium nitroprusside is contained in 250 ml of D_5W?*

Step 1:

$$mg / ml = \frac{mg \text{ of drug}}{ml \text{ of IV fluids}}$$

$$concentration = \frac{50 \text{ mg}}{250 \text{ ml}}$$

concentration = 0.2 mg/ml

Step 2:
Convert from milligrams per milliliter to micrograms per milliliter using the factor (1000 mcg = 1 mg) (See Appendix G):

$$\frac{0.2 \text{ mg}}{1 \text{ ml}} \times \frac{1000 \text{ mcg}}{1 \text{ mg}} = \frac{200 \text{ mcg}}{1 \text{ ml}}$$

When precision is required, such as in the mixing of emergency drugs, an equal volume of solution should be removed prior to adding the drug, or the volume of the drug should be incorporated into the equation as in the example above.

★ **Example:** *If you need to give 10 mcg/kg/minute of sodium nitroprusside to a 10 kg dog to maintain blood pressure, how many drops/minute should you give using a 60-drop set (e.g., 60 gtt = 1 ml)?*

Step 1:
dose (mcg/min) = dosage (mcg/kg/min) × wt (kg)

dose = 10 mcg/kg/min × 10 kg

dose = 100 mg/min

Step 2:
Divide the dose needed in mcg/min (100 mcg/min) in the previous example by the concentration of the nitroprusside (200 mcg/ml) to obtain the required volume per minute:

$$\text{volume (ml)} = \frac{\text{dose (mcg / min)}}{\text{concentration (mcg / ml)}}$$

$$\text{volume} = \frac{100 \text{ mcg / min}}{200 \text{ mcg / ml}}$$

volume = 0.5 ml/min

Step 3:
Since a 60-drop (microdrip) set has 60 drops (gtt) per milliliter, multiply the desired rate (ml/min) by the number of drops per milliliter to determine the number of drops per minute required to administer 10 mg/kg/min:

drops/minute = rate (ml/min) × drops/ml

drops/minute = 60 gtt/ml × 0.5 ml/minute

drops/minute = **30 drops/minute**

★ **Example:** *Heparin is often used to help keep catheters patent. Heparin flush is usually a 10 U/ml solution. If large amounts of heparin flush are being required, such as in ICU or anesthesia preparation areas, a liter may be prepared and individual doses drawn up in anticipation of* *need. How much 1000 U/ml heparin should be added to 1L of 0.9% NaCl to make the resulting solution 10 U/ml?*

Step 1:

volume × concentration = volume × concentration

Convert liters to milliliters (See Appendix G):

$$1 \, L \times \frac{1000 \, ml}{L} = 1000 \, ml$$

unknown ml × 1000 U/ml = 10 U / ml × 1000 ml

$$\text{unknown ml} = \frac{10 \, \cancel{U} / \cancel{ml} \times 1000 \, ml}{1000 \, \cancel{U} / \cancel{ml}}$$

unknown ml = **10 ml**

Step 2:

Add 10 ml of 1000 U/ml heparin to 1 liter of NaCl to make a liter of 10 U/ml.

Alternate Method:

The amount of heparin required could have been calculated by:

$$\frac{10 \, U}{1 \, \cancel{ml}} \times \frac{1000 \, \cancel{ml}}{1 \, L} = \frac{10,000 \, U}{L}$$

Then the volume of 1000 U/ml heparin calculated:

$$\text{required ml} = \frac{10,000 \, U}{1000 \, U / ml}$$

required ml = **10 ml**

★ **Example:** *To administer heparin at a therapeutic dose of 80 U/hour using a 10 U/ml solution, how should the IVAC pump be set in ml/hr?*

$$\text{rate (ml / hr)} = \frac{\text{concentration / hr}}{\text{concentration / ml}}$$

$$\text{rate} = \frac{80 \text{ U / hr}}{10 \text{ U / ml}}$$

$$\text{rate} = \frac{8 \text{ ml}}{1 \text{ hr}}$$

★ **Example:** *A goat is to receive 750 ml of fluids per day. a) How many milliliters per hour and b) how many milliliters per minute should the goat receive?*

a) To calculate the milliliters per hour, divide the volume (ml) by the duration of therapy (hours):

$$\text{ml / hr} = \frac{\text{dose (ml)}}{\text{\# of hours}}$$

$$\text{ml / hr} = \frac{750 \text{ ml}}{24 \text{ hr}}$$

ml/hr = **31.25 ml / hr**

b) To calculate milliliters per minute, divide the milliliters per hour by 60 minutes per hour:

$$\text{ml / min} = \frac{\text{ml / hr}}{60 \text{ min / hr}}$$

$$\text{ml / min} = \frac{31.25 \text{ ml / hr}}{60 \text{ min / hr}}$$

ml/min = **0.52 ml / min**

Using a microdrop set (60 drops/ml) the drip rate for this patient should be

$$\text{drip rate} = \frac{\text{ml required}}{\text{time}} \times \frac{\text{drops}}{1 \text{ ml}}$$

$$\text{drip rate} = \frac{0.52 \text{ ml}}{1 \text{ min}} \times \frac{60 \text{ drops}}{1 \text{ ml}}$$

drip rate = **31.2 drops / min**

★ **Example:** *A horse is to receive 10 L of lactated Ringer's solution (LRS) during 12 hr. Determine the drip rate using a set that delivers 10 gtt/ml.*

$$\text{drip rate} = \frac{\text{ml required}}{\text{time}} \times \frac{\text{drops}}{1 \text{ ml}}$$

Step 1:
Convert the volume to be administered from liters to milliliters (See Appendix G):

$$\frac{10 \text{ L}}{12 \text{ hr}} \times \frac{1000 \text{ ml}}{1 \text{ L}} = \frac{10,000 \text{ ml}}{12 \text{ hr}}$$

Step 2:
Convert the time from hours to minutes:

$$\frac{10,000 \text{ ml}}{12 \text{ hr}} \times \frac{1 \text{ hr}}{60 \text{ min}} = 13.889 \text{ ml / min}$$

Step 3:
Determine the number of gtt/min using an administering set that delivers 10 gtt/ml:

$$\frac{13.889 \text{ ml}}{1 \text{ min}} \times \frac{10 \text{ gtt}}{1 \text{ ml}} \approx 139 \text{ gtt / min}$$

Alternate Method for Steps 1 to 3:
For steps 1 to 3:

$$\text{drip rate} = \frac{10 \cancel{\text{L}} \times (1000 \text{ ml} / \cancel{\text{L}})}{12 \cancel{\text{hours}} \times (60 \text{ min} / \cancel{\text{hr}})} \times \frac{10 \text{ drops}}{1 \text{ ml}}$$

$$\text{drip rate} = \frac{10,000 \cancel{\text{ml}}}{720 \text{ min}} \times \frac{10 \text{ drops}}{1 \cancel{\text{ml}}}$$

$$\text{drip rate} = \frac{100,000 \text{ drops}}{720 \text{ min}}$$

drip rate = 138.889 ≈ **139 drops / min**

★ **Example:** *A dog is to receive 1 g of theophylline in 500 ml of LRS during 24 hr. a) What is the hourly dose of theophylline? b) How many milliliters should be administered?*

$$\text{a) dose / hr} = \frac{\text{mg of drug} \times \text{flow rate (ml / hr)}}{\text{ml of solution}}$$

$$\text{dose / hr} = \frac{1000 \text{ mg} \times (500 \cancel{\text{ml}} / 24 \text{ hr})}{500 \cancel{\text{ml}}}$$

dose/hr = **42 mg / hr of theophylline**

$$\text{b) ml / hr} = \frac{500 \text{ ml}}{24 \text{ hr}}$$

ml/hr = 20.8 or ≈ **21 ml / hr**

★ **Example:** *A 350 g Amazon parrot is to receive 8.75 mg of doxycyline I.V. through an intraosseous cannula. The solution is to be delivered slowly during 45 minutes. What is the drip rate per minute if the doxycycline is diluted in 10 ml of normal saline (0.9% NaCl)?*

$$\text{rate (ml / min)} = \frac{10 \text{ ml}}{45 \text{ min}} = 0.22 \text{ ml / min}$$

$$\text{rate (mg / min)} = \frac{8.75 \text{ mg}}{45 \text{ min}} = 0.19 \text{ mg / min}$$

Practice Problems
(See Appendix H for answers)

94. Dopamine is prescribed at 5 mcg/kg/min for a 40 lb dog. What should the rate be in milliliters per hour if dopamine is available as an 800 mg in 500 ml solution?

95. How many drops per minute are needed to deliver 8 ml/hour using a pediatric drip set (60 drops/ml)?

96. If a horse is receiving 210 drops/min of an isotonic bicarb solution using a drip set that delivers 15 drops/ml, how long will it take to administer 10 L of the solution?

97. Gentamicin (60 mg) is diluted in 50 ml of solution to be infused during 30 minutes. What should the pump rate be in ml/hour?

98. How much U-100 regular insulin is needed to make a 1 U/ml insulin drip in 250 ml normal saline (0.9% NaCl)?

99. If the insulin drip in question number 98 is to be infused at 6 ml/hr, how much insulin will be delivered in 24 hours?

100. What is the mg/ml concentration of 1:1000 epinephrine?

Parts per Million (ppm)

Parts per million (ppm) is defined as the number of parts of solute contained in one million parts of solution. That is, part per million is 1 g solute in one million milliliters, or 1 g in 264 gallons, or 1 g in 35.3 cubic feet. (1 ppm = 1 part / 10^6 = 1 g / 264 gal = 1 g / 35.3 ft^3)

Converting Parts per Million to Gallons

★ **Example:** *If a bucket holds 20 gallons, how much iodine must be added to make a concentration of 1 ppm?*

Step 1:

Convert from gallons to milliliters using the fact that 1 gallon contains 3,785 ml (See Appendix G):

$$\frac{20 \text{ gal}}{1} \times \frac{3,785 \text{ ml}}{1 \text{ gal}} = 75,700 \text{ ml}$$

Step 2:

Set up a ratio to determine how many grams are contained in 75,700 ml if 1 g is contained in 1,000,000 ml:

$$\frac{1 \text{ g}}{1,000,000 \text{ ml}} = \frac{\text{unknown g}}{75,700 \text{ ml}}$$

Cross multiply to solve the equation:

$$\text{unknown g} \times 1,000,000 = 1 \times 75,700$$

$$\text{unknown g} = \frac{75,700}{1,000,000}$$

$$\text{unknown g} = 0.0757 \text{ g}$$

$$\text{mg} = 0.0757 \text{ g} \times \frac{1000 \text{ mg}}{1 \text{ g}}$$

$$\text{mg} = 75.7 \text{ mg} \approx \textbf{76 mg}$$

★ **Example:** *Make a 200 ppm solution from a 1 quart stock solution that is 2%.*

By convention, percentage (%) = g/100 ml, so 2% = 2 g/100 ml.

Step 1:

Set up a ratio to express the concentration of the stock solution in parts per million (ppm) :

$$\frac{2 \text{ g}}{100 \text{ ml}} = \frac{\text{unknown ppm}}{1,000,000 \text{ ml}}$$

Cross multiply to solve the equation:

unknown ppm × 100 = 2 × 1,000,000

$$\text{unknown ppm} = \frac{2,000,000}{100}$$

unknown ppm = 20,000 ppm

Step 2:
Use the equation (concentration × volume = concentration × volume) to determine how much of a 200 ppm solution can be made from the 1 quart (946 ml) of 20,000 ppm stock solution:

concentration × volume = concentration × volume

20,000 ppm × 946 ml = 200 ppm × required vol

18,920,000 = 200 × required volume

$$\frac{18,920,000}{200} = \text{required volume}$$

94,600 ml = required volume

Step 3:
That is, 1 quart of a 2% (20,000 ppm) solution will make 94,600 ml of a 200 ppm solution. Since there are 3,785 ml/gallon, how many gallons can be made?

$$\frac{94.600 \text{ ml}}{3,785 \text{ ml / gal}} = 24.99 \text{ gallons} \approx 25 \text{ gallons}$$

Thus, 1 quart of a 2% (20,000 ppm) solution will make almost 25 gallons of a 200 ppm solution.

Step 4:
To make a single gallon of a 200 ppm solution from the 20,000 ppm stock solution set up the following equation:

concentration × volume = concentration × volume

200 ppm × unknown ml = 200 ppm × 3,785

$$\text{unknown ml} = \frac{200 \times 3,785}{20,000}$$

unknown ml = 37.85 ml ≈ **38 ml**

Approximately 38 ml of a 2% (20,000 ppm) solution will make one gallon of 200 ppm solution. Since this volume will be contained in the gallon, only 3,747 ml of water or other suitable diluent will be needed to make 1 gallon of a 200 ppm solution (3,785 ml – 38 ml = 3,747 ml).

★ **Example:** *If you need a farmer to treat a herd of calves with a coccidiostat in the drinking water at a rate of 1 oz per gallon and the farmer has a 250 gallon water tank, how much coccidiostat must be added?*

1 oz / gal × 250 gal = 250 oz of coccidiostat needed

Since each gallon contains 128 oz, we can convert to a more easily measured unit (gallons) (See Appendix G):

$$\text{gal} = 250 \, \cancel{oz} \times \frac{1 \text{ gal}}{128 \, \cancel{oz}}$$

gal = 1.98 gallons or ≈ 2 gallons of coccidiostat should be added to the 250 gallon tank.

What is the final concentration of coccidiostat in ppm if the original concentration of coccidiostat was 9.6%?

Step 1:
Determine the number of grams that will be contained in 1 oz of stock solution. Each ounce contains 29.57 ml. (This is often rounded off to 30 ml.) (See Appendix G)

To determine the number of grams that will be contained in 1 oz of stock solution, convert the original concentration from a percentage to grams. This can be done using the fact that % = g/100 ml.

$$9.6\% = \frac{9.6 \text{ g}}{100 \text{ ml}}$$

$$\frac{9.6 \text{ g}}{100 \cancel{\text{ ml}}} \times \frac{30 \cancel{\text{ ml}}}{1 \text{ oz}} = 2.88 \text{ g/oz}$$

Step 2:
Since 2.88 g will be diluted in each gallon of drinking water, a ratio can be set up to determine the ppm of the resulting solution using the fact that 1 gallon contains 3,785 ml and ppm is defined as grams per 10^6 ml:

$$\frac{2.88 \text{ g}}{3,785 \text{ ml}} = \frac{\text{unknown g}}{1,000,000 \text{ ml}}$$

Cross multiply to solve the equation.

$$\text{unknown} \times 3,785 = 2.88 \times 1,000,000$$

$$\text{unknown} = \frac{2.8 \times 1,000,000}{3,785}$$

$$\text{unknown} = \frac{2,880,000}{3,785}$$

$$\text{unknown} = \textbf{761 ppm}$$

The final solution contains 761 ppm of coccidiostat.

★ **Example:** *Metronidazole can be used to treat ick in a household aquarium at a dose of 250 mg per tank. What is the ppm concentration if the tank is a) 10 gallons, b) 20 gallons, or c) 40 gallons?*

a) To determine the ppm, common units must be established. Convert from milligrams per tank to grams per gallon. In this case use a tank size of 10 gallons.

$$\frac{250 \text{ mg}}{10 \text{ gal}} \times \frac{1 \text{ g}}{1000 \text{ mg}} = 0.025 \text{ g / gal}$$

Next convert from gallons to milliliters using the fact that 1 gallon = 3,785 ml (See Appendix G):

$$\frac{0.025 \text{ g}}{1 \text{ gal}} \times \frac{1 \text{ gal}}{3,785 \text{ ml}} = \frac{0.025 \text{ g}}{3,785 \text{ ml}}$$

Set up a ratio using the definition of ppm = $g/10^6$ ml:

$$\frac{0.025 \text{ g}}{3,785 \text{ ml}} = \frac{\text{unknown g}}{1,000,000 \text{ ml}}$$

Cross multiply to solve the equation:

unknown × 3,785 = 0.025 × 1,000,000

$$\text{unknown} = \frac{0.025 \times 1,000,000}{3,785}$$

unknown = **6.6 ppm**

b) To convert from milligrams/tank to ppm, first convert to grams/gallon using a 20 gallon tank:

$$\frac{250 \text{ mg}}{20 \text{ gal}} \times \frac{1 \text{ g}}{1000 \text{ mg}} = 0.0125 \text{ g / gallon}$$

Next convert from gallons to milliliters using the fact that 1 gallon = 3,785 ml (See Appendix G):

$$\frac{0.0125 \text{ g}}{1 \text{ gal}} \times \frac{1 \text{ gal}}{3,785 \text{ ml}} = \frac{0.0125 \text{ g}}{3,785 \text{ ml}}$$

Set up a ratio using the definition of ppm = $g/10^6$ ml:

$$\frac{0.0125 \text{ g}}{3,785 \text{ ml}} = \frac{\text{unknown g}}{1,000,000 \text{ ml}}$$

Cross multiply to solve the equation:

unknown × 3,785 = 0.0125 × 1,000,000

$$\text{unknown} = \frac{0.0125 \times 1,000,000}{3,785}$$

unknown = **3.3 ppm**

c) To convert from mg/40 gallon tank to ppm first convert to grams per gallon:

$$\frac{250 \text{ mg}}{40 \text{ gal}} \times \frac{1 \text{ g}}{1000 \text{ mg}} = 0.006 \text{ g / gal}$$

Next convert from gallons to milliliters using the fact that 1 gallon = 3,785 ml:

$$\frac{0.006 \text{ g}}{1 \text{ gal}} \times \frac{1 \text{ gal}}{3,785 \text{ ml}} = \frac{0.006 \text{ g}}{3,785}$$

Set up a ratio using the definition of ppm = $g/10^6$ ml:

$$\frac{0.006 \text{ g}}{3,785 \text{ ml}} = \frac{\text{unknown g}}{1,000,000 \text{ ml}}$$

Cross multiply to solve the equation:

unknown × 3,785 = 0.006 × 1,000,000

$$\text{unknown} = \frac{0.006 \times 1,000,000}{3,785}$$

unknown = **1.58 ppm**

Converting Parts per Million to Grams per Cubic Foot

★ **Example:** *An antimicrobial has been recommended by a microbiologist to treat catfish in a commercial setting. If the recommended dose is 10 ppm, how many grams will be required to treat the breeder pool (250,000 ft³ of water)?*

Step 1:
By convention,
1 ppm = 0.028 g/ft³

To determine how many g/ft³ are required to make 10 ppm set up a ratio:

$$\frac{1\ \text{ppm}}{10\ \text{ppm}} = \frac{0.028\ \text{g} / \text{ft}^3}{\text{unknown g} / \text{ft}^3}$$

Cross multiply to solve the equation:

unknown g/ft³ × 1 = 0.028 × 10

unknown g/ft³ = 0.28 g/ft³

Step 2:
To determine the number of grams of the antimicrobial needed to treat the tank, multiply the dose required (0.28 g/ft³) by the volume of the tank (250,000 ft³):

dose (g) = concentration (g/ft³) × volume (ft³)

$$\text{dose} = \frac{0.28\ \text{g}}{1\ \cancel{\text{ft}^3}} \times 250,000\ \cancel{\text{ft}^3}$$

dose = 70,000 g

Step 3:

For more convenient measurements, the result could then be converted to kilograms (1 kg = 1000 g) (See Appendix G):

$$\frac{70,000 \cancel{g}}{1} \times \frac{1 \text{ kg}}{1000 \cancel{g}} = 70 \text{ kg}$$

or pounds (1 lb = 454 g)

$$\frac{70,000 \cancel{g}}{1} \times \frac{1 \text{ lb}}{454 \cancel{g}} = 154.2 \text{ lb}$$

Converting Parts per Million to Grams per Milliliter, Milligrams per Milliliter, and a Percentage

★ **Example:** *Convert 10,000 ppm to a) g/ml, b) mg/ml, and c) a percentage.*

a) To convert from ppm to g/ml, use the fact that ppm = $g/10^6$ ml and reduce to lowest terms.

$$10,000 \text{ ppm} = \frac{10,000 \text{ g}}{1,000,000 \text{ ml}} = \frac{1 \text{ g}}{100 \text{ ml}} = \frac{0.01 \text{ g}}{\text{ml}}$$

b) Convert ppm from $g/10^6$ ml to mg/ml by multiplying by the conversion factor 1 g = 1000 mg and then reducing it to the lowest terms.

$$10,000 \text{ ppm} = \frac{10,000 \cancel{g}}{1,000,000 \text{ ml}} \times \frac{1000 \text{ mg}}{1 \cancel{g}} = \frac{10 \text{ mg}}{\text{ml}}$$

c) To convert from ppm to a percentage, recall that % = g/100 ml. Set up a ratio using the fact that ppm = g/1,000,000 ml and % = g/100 ml:

$$\frac{10,000 \text{ g}}{1,000,000 \text{ ml}} = \frac{\text{unknown g}}{100 \text{ ml}}$$

Cross multiply to solve the equation.

unknown × 1,000,000 = 10,000 × 100

$$\text{unknown} = \frac{10,000 \times 100}{1,000,000}$$

unknown = 1%

Practice Problems
(See Appendix H for answers)

101. How many ppm would a 0.5% solution be?
102. How many grams of sodium bicarbonate should be added to 1 gal of water to make a 100 ppm solution?
103. How much of a 2% NaOH is needed to make 1 L of a 100 ppm buffer solution?
104. How much metronidazole is needed to treat a 250 gal tank at 6 ppm? Metronidazole is available in 250 mg and 500 mg tablets.
105. Sodium acetate is commercially available as a 40 mEq/20 ml solution that contains 164 mg of sodium acetate anhydrous/ml. What is the concentration in ppm of the commercial preparation?

Percentages

By definition, % = g/100 ml, so 0.01% = 0.01 g/ml = 10 mg/ml. In solutions or mixtures, percentage concentration may be expressed as: percentage weight in weight (w/w), percentage weight in volume (w/v), or percentage volume in volume (v/v).

Weight / Weight

Percentage weight in weight (w/w) expresses the number of grams of a solute in 100 g of solution. Examples of weight preparations are a 1% hydrocortisone ointment that contains 1 g hydrocortisone in each 100 g of ointment or a 20% salicyclic acid poultice containing 20 g of salicyclic acid in each 100 g of paste.

★ **Example**: *To manufacture BIPP ointment, 454 of iodoform powder are mixed with 227 g of bismuth subnitrate and incorporated into 8 oz of petrolatum paste. Determine the resulting percentage (w/w) of a) bismuth, b) petrolatum, and c) iodoform powder by dividing the weight of the constituent part by the sum of the total weight of the parts:*

a) % bismuth subnitrate (w/w) = wt bismuth × 100%
   wt of BIPP

wt of BIPP = 227 g bismuth + 454 g iodoform powder

$$+ \ 8 \ \text{oz petrolatum} \times \frac{28.35 \ \text{g}}{1 \ \text{oz}}$$

weight of BIPP = 227 g + 454 g + 226.8 g

weight of BIPP = 907.8

$$\% \ \text{of bismuth subnitrate} = \frac{\text{wt of bismuth}}{\text{wt of BIPP}} \times 100\%$$

$$\% \ = \frac{227 \ \text{g}}{907.8} \times 100\%$$

% bismuth = **25%**

b) $\% \ \text{petrolatum} \ (w/w) = \dfrac{\text{wt petrolatum}}{\text{wt of BIPP}} \times 100\%$

$$\% \ = \frac{\text{wt petrolatum}}{\text{wt of BIPP}} \times 100\%$$

$$\% = \frac{226.8}{907.8} \times 100\%$$

% petrolatum = **25%**

c) % iodoform powder $= \dfrac{\text{wt of iodoform powder}}{\text{wt of BIPP}} \times 100\%$

$$\% = \frac{454\ g}{907.8} \times 100\%$$

% iodoform = **50%**

*Note: If the sum of percentages of the individual compo-
nents does not add up to 100%, an error has been made
in the calculation.*

Weight / Volume

Percentage weight in volume (w/v) expresses the number of grams (weight) of constituent or solute in 100
ml of solution (volume). Examples of weight in volume
preparations are a 2% (w/v) sodium solution that contains 2 g of sodium (Na) in 100 ml of solution or a
50% (w/v) dextrose solution that contains 50 g of dextrose in 100 ml of solution.

★ **Example:** *After constitution, what is the (w/v) percentage for Amoxidrops® in a 50 mg/ml suspension?*

Step 1:
Convert the concentration from mg/ml to g/ml.

$$\text{unknown} = \frac{50\ \cancel{mg}}{ml} \times \frac{1\ g}{1000\ \cancel{mg}}$$

$$\text{unknown} = \frac{50\ g}{1000\ ml}$$

unknown = 0.05 g/ml

Step 2:

Set up a ratio using the fact that % = g/100 ml:

$$\frac{0.05\ g}{1\ ml} = \frac{unknown\ g}{100\ ml}$$

Cross multiply to solve the equation.

unknown × 1 = 0.05 × 100

unknown = 5%

Volume / Volume

Percentage volume in volume (v/v) expresses the number of milliliters of a solute in 100 ml of solution. Examples of volume in volume preparations are a 10% (v/v) Clorox® solution containing 10 ml of Clorox® in 100 ml of solution or a 70% (v/v) ethyl alcohol solution containing 70 ml of ethyl alcohol in 100 ml of solution.

★ **Example:** *Nolvasan® solution is available commercially as a 2% solution, but a 0.05% solution is recommended for flushing wounds. How much Nolvasan 2% solution should be added to 1 L of water before flushing wounds? [Remember Nolvasan® is incompatible with electrolyte solutions like 0.9% NaCl, Ringer's, or lactated Ringer's solution].*

Step 1:

To make 1 liter (1000 ml) of a 0.05% solution using a 2% stock solution use the equation:

concentration × volume = concentration × volume

2% × unknown volume = 0.05% × 100 ml

$$\text{unknown volume} = \frac{0.05\% \times 100 \text{ ml}}{2\%}$$

unknown volume = 25 ml

The addition of 25 ml of Nolvasan® to 1000 ml of sterile water will make approximately a 0.05% (0.0488%) flush. To determine exactly how much Nolvasan® solution would be required, an equal volume of water (25 ml) must be removed prior to the addition of Nolvasan®, or the volume of the Nolvasan® must be considered in the equation thus:

concentration × volume = concentration × volume

2% × unknown volume = 0.05% × (1 L + Vol. Nolvasan®)

2% × unknown volume = 0.05% × (1000 ml + unknown volume)

2 × unknown volume = 50 ml + 0.05 unknown volume

1.95 unknown volume = 50 ml

unknown volume = **25.6 ml**

To make precisely a 0.05% solution, 25.6 ml of Nolvasan® should be added to 1000 ml of water. When precision is required such as in the mixing of emergency drugs, an equal volume of solution should be removed prior to adding the drug, or the volume of the drug should be incorporated into the equation as in the example above.

Converting Percentages to Milligrams or Micrograms

★ **Example**: *Ivermectin is an abamectin used to control a variety of parasites in animals. To treat a*

35 lb dog (not a collie) with a microfilarcide dose of ivermectin (50 mcg/kg), how much of the commercial 1% preparation will you need?

Step 1:
Convert the dog's weight from pounds to kilograms (See Appendix G):

$$\text{wt in kg} = \frac{\text{wt (lb)}}{1} \times \frac{1 \text{ kg}}{2.2 \text{ lb}}$$

$$\text{wt in kg} = \frac{35 \text{ lb}}{1} \times \frac{1 \text{ kg}}{2.2 \text{ lb}} = 15.9 \text{ kg}$$

Step 2:
Multiply the dose (50 mcg/kg) by the animal's weight (kg):

$$\text{dose (mcg)} = \frac{\text{dose mcg}}{1 \text{ kg}} \times \frac{\text{wt (kg)}}{1}$$

$$\text{dose} = \frac{50 \text{ mcg}}{1 \text{ kg}} \times \frac{15.9 \text{ kg}}{1}$$

dose = 795 mcg

Step 3:
Convert the commercial preparation from a percentage to mg/ml recalling that % = g/100 ml:

$$1\% = \frac{1 \text{ g}}{100 \text{ ml}} = \frac{1000 \text{ mg}}{100 \text{ ml}} = \frac{10 \text{ mg}}{\text{ml}}$$

$$\frac{10 \text{ mg}}{\text{ml}} \times \frac{1000 \text{ mcg}}{1 \text{ mg}} = 10,000 \text{ mcg / ml}$$

Step 4:
Determine the volume required to supply the dose of 759 micrograms:

$$dose = \frac{795 \text{ mcg}}{1} \times \frac{1 \text{ ml}}{10,000 \text{ mcg}}$$

dose = 0.00795 ml ≈ **0.08 ml**

★ **Example:** *To treat the same 35 lb dog for round-worms with a dose of 200 mcg of ivermectin per kilogram of body weight, how much of the commercial 1% preparation would you need to use?*

Step 1:
Convert the weight from pounds to kilograms (See Appendix G):

$$\text{wt in kg} = \frac{\text{wt in lb}}{1} \times \frac{1 \text{ kg}}{2.2 \text{ lb}}$$

$$\text{wt in kg} = \frac{35 \text{ lb}}{1} \times \frac{1 \text{ kg}}{2.2 \text{ lb}} = 15.9 \text{ kg}$$

Step 2:
Multiply the animal's weight (kg) by the dose required in micrograms per kilogram:

$$\text{dose in mcg} = \frac{\text{dose (mcg)}}{1 \text{ kg}} \times \frac{\text{wt in kilograms}}{1}$$

$$\text{dose} = \frac{200 \text{ mcg}}{1 \text{ kg}} \times \frac{15.9 \text{ kg}}{1}$$

$$\text{dose} = \frac{3,180 \text{ mcg}}{1} \times \frac{1 \text{ mg}}{1000 \text{ mcg}}$$

dose = **3.18 mg**

Step 3:
Convert the concentration of the commercial prepara-tion from a percentage to mg/ml:

$$1\% = \frac{1 \text{ g}}{100 \text{ ml}}$$

$$\text{concentration} = \frac{1 \cancel{g}}{100 \text{ ml}} \times \frac{1000 \text{ mg}}{1 \cancel{g}}$$

$$\text{concentration} = \frac{1000 \text{ mg}}{100 \text{ ml}}$$

concentration = 10 mg/ml

Step 4:
To determine the volume required, set up a ratio:

$$\frac{3.18 \text{ mg}}{10 \text{ mg}} = \frac{\text{unknown ml}}{1 \text{ ml}}$$

Cross multiply to solve the equation:

unknown ml × 10 = 3.18 × 1

$$\text{unknown ml} = \frac{3.18}{10} = 0.318 \text{ ml} \approx 0.32 \text{ ml}$$

Converting Percentages to Milliequivalents

★ **Example:** *How many milliequivalents of magnesium are in 10 ml of 50% magnesium sulfate (MgSO₄) injection?*

$$\text{mEq} = \frac{g \times 1000}{\text{mw}} \times \text{valence}$$

Step 1:
Determine the number of grams of magnesium sulfate contained in 10 ml of the 50% solution:

$$\% = \frac{1 \text{ g}}{100 \text{ ml}}$$

$$50\% = \frac{50 \text{ g}}{100 \text{ ml}}$$

50% = 5 g/10 ml

Step 2:
Determine the molecular weight of magnesium sulfate (See Appendix D):

mw of $MgSO_4 \bullet 7H_2O = mwMg^{+2} + mwSO_4^{-2} + mw7H_2O$

mw $MgSO_4 \bullet 7H_2O = 24.3 + [32.06 + (4 \times 15.99)] + 7 \times [(2 \times 1) + 15.99]$

mw $MgSO_4 \bullet 7H_2O = 246$

Step 3:
Substituting into the milliequivalent equation, determine the number of mEq/10 ml:

$MgSO_4 \bullet 7H_2O = mwMg^{+2} + mwSO_4^{-2} + mw7H_2O$

The valence of Mg is 2.

Substituting the known values into the equation:

$$\frac{mEq}{10\ ml} = \frac{g \times 1000}{mw} \times valence$$

$$\frac{mEq}{10\ ml} = \frac{5 \times 1000}{246} \times 2$$

Thus, there are **40.6 mEq / 10 ml**

★ **Example:** *A vial of sodium chloride (NaCl) injection contains 4 mEq/ml. What is the percent strength of this solution?*

Since percent is defined as grams per 100 milliliters, we need to determine the number of grams of NaCl contained in 100 ml.

$$mEq = \frac{g \times 1000}{mw} \times valence$$

Step 1:
Determine the valence of NaCl (See Appendix D):

$NaCl = Na^+ Cl^-$

The valence is 1.

Step 2:
Determine the molecular weight of NaCl
(See Appendix D):

mw NaCl = mw Na^+ + mw Cl^-
mw NaCl = 23 + 35.5
mw NaCl = 58.5

Substitute the known values into the equation:

$$\frac{4 \text{ mEq}}{1 \text{ ml}} = \frac{\text{mw NaCl g} \times 1000}{58.5} \times 1$$

Cross multiply to solve for mw NaCl:

$4 \times 58.5 =$ mw NaCl $\times 1000 \times 1$
$234 =$ mw NaCl $\times 1000$

$$\text{mw NaCl} = \frac{234}{1000}$$

mw NaCl = 0.234 g/ml

Step 3:
Convert from g/ml to g/100 ml to find the percentage:

$$\frac{0.234 \text{ g}}{\text{ml}} = \frac{\text{mw NaCl}}{100 \text{ ml}}$$

Cross multiply to solve the equation.

mw NaCl = 23.4 g/100 ml

Then, substitute into the equation:

$$\% = \frac{g}{100 \text{ ml}}$$

$$\% = \frac{23.4 \text{ g}}{100 \text{ ml}}$$

$$\% = 23.4\%$$

Milligram Percent

Milligram percent (mg %) is the number of milligrams of a substance in 100 ml of liquid. It is often used to denote the concentration of a drug or natural substance in body fluids like blood or plasma.

★ **Example:** *Magnesium (Mg) levels in the blood are determined to be 2.5 mEq/L. What is the mg percentage?*

Step 1:
Determine the number of mEq of magnesium found in 100 ml of blood by using the ratio

$$\frac{\text{unknown mEq}}{2.5 \text{ mEq}} = \frac{100 \text{ ml}}{1000 \text{ ml}}$$

Cross multiply to solve the equation.

$$\text{unknown mEq} = \frac{2.5 \times 100}{1000}$$

$$\text{unknown mEq} = 0.25 \text{ mEq}$$

Step 2:
To convert milliequivalents (mEq) to milligrams (mg), recall that:

$$\text{mEq} = \frac{\text{mg}}{\text{mw}} \times \text{valence}$$

Therefore,

$$\frac{mEq}{100ml} = \frac{mg/100 \ ml}{mw} \times valence$$

From Appendix D, obtain the molecular weight (mw) of magnesium (Mg) and its valence and substitute into the equation:

$$\frac{0.25 \ mEq}{100 \ ml} = \frac{mg/100 \ ml}{mw} \times valence$$

$$\frac{0.25 \ mEq}{100 \ ml} = \frac{mg/100 \ ml}{24.3} \times 2$$

$$\left(\frac{0.25 \ mEq}{100 \ ml}\right) \times 24.3 = 2 \times \left(\frac{mg}{100 \ ml}\right)$$

$$\frac{6.07}{100 \ ml} = 2 \times \frac{mg}{100 \ ml}$$

$$\frac{mg}{100 \ ml} = \frac{6.07 \ / \ 100 \ ml}{2}$$

$$\frac{mg}{100 \ ml} = \frac{3.03}{100 \ ml}$$

Therefore,

$$\frac{0.25 \ mEq}{100 \ ml} = \frac{2.5 \ mEq}{1 \ L} = 3.03 \ mg\%$$

Percentage of Error

Percentage of error determines the limitations of instruments of measure (such as a tension balance, beaker, or graduated cylinder) and the error that may be incurred when using them.

$$\text{percentage of error} = \frac{\text{error} \times 100\%}{\text{measured quantity}}$$

This equation can also be used to calculate the least amount that can be weighed.

★ **Example**: *If a torsion balance has a sensitivity of 1/16 grain, what is the smallest amount that can be weighed with a potential error of not more than 2%?*

$$\text{percentage of error} = \frac{\text{error} \times 100\%}{\text{quantity desired}}$$

$$2\% = \frac{\dfrac{1}{16\ \text{gr}} \times \dfrac{100\%}{1}}{\text{quantity desired}}$$

$$\text{quantity desired} \times 2 = \frac{100}{16}\ \text{gr}$$

quantity desired × 2 = 6.25 gr

$$\text{quantity desired} = \frac{6.25\ \text{gr}}{2}$$

quantity desired = 3.125 gr = **3 1/8 grains**

Thus, 3 1/8 grains is the least amount that can be weighed accurately on the balance.

★ **Example**: *If a 98% accuracy is desired, what is the minimum amount that should be weighed on a torsion prescription balance having a sensitivity of 0.004 g?*

Step 1:
100% – 98% accuracy = 2% error

Step 2:

$$\text{percentage of error} = \frac{\text{error} \times 100\%}{\text{quantity desired}}$$

$$2\% = \frac{0.004 \times 100\%}{\text{quantity desired}}$$

$$2 \times \text{quantity desired} = 0.4 \text{ g}$$

$$\text{quantity desired} = \frac{0.4 \text{ g}}{2}$$

$$\text{quantity desired} = \textbf{0.2 g}$$

Thus, 0.2 g is the least amount that can be weighed accurately on this balance.

★ **Example:** *If you measure 900 ml in a 1000 ml graduated cylinder that is calibrated in units of 10 ml, what is the percentage of error that might be incurred in this measurement?*

Since the graduation can accurately be measured in units of 10 ml, 10 ml is the sensitivity of the cylinder, or the amount of error that may be obtained in the measurement. Substitute this into the equation:

$$\% \text{ error} = \frac{\text{error} \times 100\%}{\text{quantity desired}}$$

$$\% \text{ error} = \frac{10 \text{ ml} \times 100\%}{900 \text{ ml}}$$

$$\% \text{ error} = \textbf{1.1\%}$$

Percentage of Alcohol

$$\text{percentage alcohol} (\%) = \frac{\text{proof strength}}{2}$$

★ **Example:** *Your formulary suggests a 10% solution of ethanol, but when your technician goes to the liquor store, he calls back to say everything is expressed in proof strength. How much 200 proof ethanol is needed to make 500 ml of a 10% solution?*

Step 1:
Convert 200 proof to percent of ethanol using the equation:

$$\% \text{ alcohol} = \frac{\text{proof strength}}{2}$$

$$\% \text{ alcohol} = \frac{200}{2}$$

% of alcohol = 100%

Step 2:
If 500 ml of 10% is needed, how much of the 100% ethanol is required?

concentration × volume = concentration × volume

100% × unknown ml = 10% × 500 ml

$$\text{unknown ml} = \frac{500 \times 10}{100}$$

unknown ml = **50 ml**

★ **Example:** *Your supplier says they can ship you 80% ethanol to arrive on Monday. What proof strength is it?*

proof strength = percent of alcohol × 2

proof strength = 80% × 2

proof strength = 160 proof

How much of this 80% ethanol would be needed to make 500 ml of 10% ethanol?

concentration × volume = concentration × volume

80% × unknown ml = 10% × 500 ml

$$\text{unknown ml} = \frac{500 \text{ ml} \times 10\%}{80\%}$$

unknown ml = **62.5 ml**

Practice Problems
(See Appendix H for answers)

106. Petercillin is a topical ointment made by warming 1 lb of lanolin and adding 1 oz of Scarlet Oil and 2 g of tetracycline. What is the final percentage of tetracycline in the preparation?
107. How many milligrams of kanamycin are required to make 250 ml of a 0.1% kanamycin irrigation solution?
108. If a 3% hydrogen peroxide solution is diluted 1:40 to clean sensitive mucous membranes, what is the resulting percentage of hydrogen peroxide?
109. How many grams of iodine are needed to make 1 pint of Lugol's solution (5% iodine solution)?
110. How many mEq of NaCl are in 500 ml of 3% sodium chloride solution?
111. A solution is listed as being slightly soluble if 1 part of solute will dissolve in 100 to 1000 parts of solvent. Substance Q is defined as slightly soluble because 1 g will dissolve in 250 ml of solvent. What is the resulting concentration of Substance Q in milligram percent (mg/100 ml)?
112. A 100 ml graduated cylinder is calibrated to deliver volumes in units of 5 ml. What is the predicted percentage of error in measuring 50 ml?

113. How much 180 proof alcohol is required to make
    1 L of D5A5 (5% dextrose + 5% alcohol)?

PNU per Milliliter

Allergens can be injected into both animals and people
at gradually increasing doses to induce an immunity.
Allergy testing reveals which antigens (e.g. weeds,
molds, trees, grasses, animals) the subject is allergic to.
Antigen solutions can be formulated to help desensi-
tize the patient to an allergen. Concentrations of the
antigen are increased depending on the patient's
response. One unit of measure used for antigen solutions is PNU (protein nitrogen units) / ml.

★ **Example:** *A dog is receiving antigens for densitiza-
    tion. How much housedust (10,000 PNU/ml),
    housedust mite (20,000 PNU/ml), and diluent
    must be added to make a 10 ml vial with a final
    concentration of 10,000 PNU/ml?*

Unless otherwise specified you would like equal concentrations (PNU/ml) of each ingredient in the final
preparation:

$$\text{volume (ml) of each antigen} = \frac{\text{total volume}}{\text{\# of antigens}}$$

$$\text{volume} = \frac{10 \text{ ml}}{2}$$

volume = **5 ml of each antigen** at a concentration of
    10,000 PNU/ml

Since housedust is already available as a 10,000
PNU/ml solution, place 5 ml of housedust in a sterile

empty vial. Housedust mite solution has a concentration of 20,000 PNU/ml. To make 5 ml of a 10,000 PNU/ml concentration of housedust mite:

volume desired × concentration desired = volume needed × original concentration

volume desired × 20,000 PNU/ ml = ml × 10,000 PNU/ml

$$\text{volume desired} = \frac{5 \text{ ml} \times 10,000 \text{ PNU / ml}}{20,000 \text{ PNU / ml}}$$

$$\text{volume desired} = \frac{50,000 \text{ ml}}{20,000}$$

volume desired = **2.5 ml**

Add 2.5 ml of housedust mite and 2.5 ml of diluent to the vial containing 5 ml of housedust. The resulting solution is 10,000 PNU/ml.

★ **Example:** *The veterinary dermatologist has written a prescription for a desensitization solution containing 60% housedust mite and 40% housedust. If housedust mite is 20,000 PNU/ml and housedust is 10,000 PNU/ml, what is the final concentration of the preparation?*

final concentration (PNU/ml) = (% × conc) + (% × conc)

final concentration =
(60% × 20,000 PNU/ml) + (40% × 10,000 PNU/ml)

final concentration =
(0.6 × 20,000 PNU/ml) + (0.4 × 10,000 PNU/ml)

final concentration = 12,000 PNU/ml + 4,000 PNU/ml

final concentration = **16,000 PNU/ml**

★ **Example:** *With skin testing, a Labrador is found to react to seven antigens. All antigens are available as 20,000 PNU/ml. To make a set of desensitizing solutions containing one 10 ml vial of 200 PNU/ml, one 10 ml vial of 2,000 PNU/ml, and one 10 ml vial containing 20,000 PNU/ml, first calculate the volume needed of each antigen:*

$$\text{volume (ml) of each antigen} = \frac{\text{total volume}}{\text{\# of antigens}}$$

$$\text{volume} = \frac{10 \text{ ml}}{7 \text{ antigens}}$$

volume = **1.43 ml of each antigen**

To make the three different concentrations, begin by making the most concentrated solution first (20,000 PNU/ml vial). Place 1.43 ml of each of the seven antigens in an empty 10 ml sterile vial. This is now a 20,000 PNU/ml vial containing all seven antigens.

To make the second vial (2,000 PNU/ml) make a 1:10 dilution of the first solution. This can be done by taking 1 ml of the 20,000 PNU/ml solution and adding 9 ml of diluent.

The third vial can be made from the second vial by making a 1:10 dilution of the second vial. That is, 1 ml of 2,000 PNU/ml is added to 9 ml of diluent.

Practice Problems
(See Appendix H for answers)

114. What volume of housedust (20,000 PNU/ml) is required to make 5 ml of a 2,000 PNU/ml solution?

115. How much housedust mite (10,000 PNU/ml) solution is required to make 10 ml of a 100 PNU/ml solution?0

116. If three antigens are to be combined to make a 5 ml preparation that is 10,000 PNU/ml, what volume of each is required if they are all 20,000 PNU/ml? How much diluent is necessary?

117. If five antigens are to be combined to make a 10 ml preparation that is 10,000 PNU/ml, what volume of each is required if they are all 20,000 PNU/ml?

118. If housedust mite (10,000 PNU/ml), mold mix (20,000 PNU/ml), and eastern tree mix (20,000 PNU/ml) are combined in equal volumes, what is the concentration of the resulting solution in PNU/ml?

Compounding

Compounding is the reformulation of an available product to a form that can be safely and accurately used to treat a specific patient. The reformulation of preparations is often required due to the variability in the size of the patients that veterinarians treat. Both parakeets and Clydesdales may benefit from ivermectin, but the dose required varies dramatically. Compounding allows the preparation of the exact dose required in a form that can be easily administered to the individual patient.

Equations

Capsules

To find the diluent required, perform the following calculations (# = number):

# of doses available =

$$\frac{\text{strength of the tablet (mg)} \times \text{\# of tablets}}{\text{\# of mg / dose}}$$

# of doses available =

$$\frac{\text{\# of capsules} \times \text{amt. of AI* per capsule}}{\text{amt. of AI* contained in each dose}}$$

total # of mg required =
(mg/dose) × (# of doses/day) × (# of days)

number or capsules needed =

$$\frac{\text{total \# of mg required}}{\text{mg per commercial capsule or tablet}}$$

$$\frac{\text{single dose}}{\text{total dose}} = \frac{\text{wt of single dose}}{\text{wt of total doses}}$$

*AI = *active ingredient*

diluent required =

$$\left[\left(\frac{\text{total amount of AI*}}{\text{amt. of AI* per dose}}\right) \times \text{wt per dose}\right] - \text{wt of AI*}$$

Oral Suspensions

total mg required =
(mg/dose) × (# of doses/day) × (# of days)

$$\text{# of capsules needed} = \frac{\text{total number of mg required}}{\text{strength of one capsule or tablet}}$$

$$\text{total volume required} = \frac{\text{total mg required}}{\text{concentration per ml}}$$

$$\frac{\text{dose desired}}{\text{volume required}} = \frac{\text{concentration}}{1\ \text{ml}}$$

Eye Drops
volume × strength = volume × strength

$$\text{ml / vial} = \frac{\text{concentration / vial}}{\text{desired concentration / ml}}$$

Topical Preparations
concentration × volume = concentration × volume

ml of commercial preparation =

$$\frac{\text{# of mg required}}{\text{concentration commercial preparation in mg / ml}}$$

Capsules

Approximate Capacity of Empty Gelatin Capsules in Grains (1 gr ≈ 65 mg) (See Appendix G):

Size	000	00	0	1	2	3	4
Lactose			8	7		4	3
Bismuth subnitrate	28	20	14	10	8	6	4
Quinine sulfate	10	6	5	3.5	3	2	1.5
Sodium bicarbonate	22	15	11	8	6	5	4
Aspirin	16	10	8	5	4	3	2.5

★ **Example**: *Phenoxybenzamine is prescribed at 0.5 mg/kg q24h for an incontinent dog. For a 5 kg dog, the calculated daily dose of phenoxybenzamine is (0.5 mg/kg q24h × 5 kg) or 2.5 mg/day. Since phenoxybenzamine is available in a 10 mg capsule and not a tablet, the 2.5 mg dose cannot be accurately obtained without reformulation. a) Determine the amount of phenoxybenzamine needed for 10 days treatment. b) Determine the number of capsules required. c) Determine if the dose can be accurately measured or if it requires reformulation. d) Reformulate the preparation.*

a) To determine the amount of phenoxybenzamine needed to treat for 10 days, multiply the dose required per day (2.5 mg) by the number of days of treatment (10):

2.5 mg/day × 10 days = **25 mg**

b) To determine the number of commercially available 10 mg capsules needed, divide the total milligrams required (25 mg, obtained in calculation a) by the concentration of one capsule (10 mg).

$$\frac{25 \text{ mg}}{10 \text{ mg / capsule}} = 2.5 \text{ capsules}$$

Since capsules can not be easily divided, use **3 capsules**. The excess can be discarded or formulated into additional dosages for later use.

c) To determine the weight of a single dose, weigh the contents of 3 capsules (30 mg of phenoxybenzamine). If the contents of 3 capsules weigh 0.624 g, how much will a single 2.5 mg dose of phenoxybenzamine weight?

$$\frac{\text{single dose}}{\text{total amount of drug}} = \frac{\text{wt of single dose}}{\text{wt of total drug}}$$

$$\frac{2.5 \text{ mg}}{3 \times 10 \text{ mg}} = \frac{\text{wt of single dose}}{0.624 \text{ g}}$$

wt of single dose × 3 × 10 mg = 2.5 mg × 0.624 g

$$\text{wt of single dose} = \frac{2.5 \text{ mg} \times 0.624 \text{ g}}{30 \text{ mg}}$$

wt of single dose = 0.092 g

The 0.092 g weight of the single or individual dose of phenoxybenzamine can be converted from grams to milligrams by multiplying the weight in grams by 1000 (See Appendix G):

$$\frac{0.092 \text{ g}}{1} \times \frac{1000 \text{ mg}}{1 \text{ g}} = 92 \text{ mg}$$

d) The use of an accurate balance is required to reformulate medications. The Class A balance is commonly used, but it is only accurate in measurements of 120 mg or more. Since 92 mg is less than 120 mg, the contents of the 3 capsules must be diluted until 2.5 mg of active ingredient is contained in an amount that you can weigh (e.g., 120 mg or more). Milk sugar or lactose is usually used. To dilute the phenoxybenzamine efficiently:

Step 1:
Take a #4 gelatin capsule and pack it with lactose. Weigh the contents, making sure that you have an empty capsule of equal size on the opposite side of the balance. This will ensure that you are weighing only the amount of lactose that is being used to fill the capsule. Most people can pack approximately 180 mg of lactose into a #4 capsule.

Step 2:
Using 180 mg as the weight contained in a #4 capsule in this example, calculate the amount of lactose that must be added to the active ingredient. To do this, first determine the number of doses that can be obtained from the 3 × 10 mg commercial capsules by multiplying the number of capsules by the amount of active ingredient contained in each capsule.

3 capsules × 10 mg/capsule = 30 mg

This calculation tells you the amount of active ingredient available for reformulation. Divide the total amount of active ingredient available by the amount of active ingredient required per dose to determine the number of doses that may be obtained from the commercial preparation.

$$\frac{30 \text{ mg}}{2.5 \text{ mg / dose}} = 12 \text{ doses}$$

These two steps can be combined into one step as shown in the equation

doses available =

$$\frac{\text{# of capsules} \times \text{amount of AI per capsule}}{\text{amount of AI contained in each dose}}$$

$$\text{doses available} = \frac{3 \text{ capsules} \times 10 \text{ mg / capsule}}{2.5 \text{ mg / dose}}$$

doses available = 12 doses

Step 3:
Determine the contents of the 12 doses by multiplying the number of doses (12) by the weight of each dose (180 mg):

total volume required = # of doses × wt of each dose

total volume = 12 doses × 180 mg/dose

total volume = 2,160 mg

Step 4:
To determine the amount of lactose required, subtract the weight of the contents of the three 10 mg capsules (0.624 g) from the total volume required. Don't forget to convert to common units:

$$\frac{2,160 \text{ mg}}{1} \times \frac{1 \text{ g}}{1000 \text{ mg}} = 2.16 \text{ g}$$

lactose required =
(total wt) – (wt of the contents of capsules)

lactose required = 2.16 g – 0.624 g
lactose required = 1.536 g ≈ **1.54 g**

Step 5:
Weigh the 1.54 g of lactose and mix it by geometric dilution (in equal parts) with the phenoxybenzamine.

Step 6:
Pack the mixture of phenoxybenzamine and lactose into #4 gelatin capsules. When you are finished there should be twelve #4 capsules each containing 180 mg (88 mg of lactose and 92 mg of phenoxybenzamine).

★ **Example:** *Oxymethalone was prescribed for your client's 26 lb dog at a dose of 15 mg orally once a day for three months. A three month supply was dispensed. You wish to continue this therapy but oxymethalone is available only as a 50 mg tablet. The owner tells you that she is running low on the capsules and needs a refill of the prescription. To make capsules containing the correct amount of oxymethalone:*

Step 1:
Calculate the number of tablets that will be required to make a three month supply. This is accomplished by multiplying the dose given per day (15 mg) by the number of days of therapy (90) and dividing the result by the strength of the commercial preparation (50 mg):

$$\text{tablets required} = \frac{\dfrac{\text{dose}}{1 \text{ day}} \times \dfrac{\text{\# of days}}{1}}{\text{tablet strength}}$$

$$\text{tablets required} = \frac{\dfrac{15 \text{ mg}}{1 \text{ day}} \times \dfrac{90 \text{ days}}{1}}{50 \text{ mg / tablet}}$$

$$\text{tablets required} = \frac{1{,}350 \text{ mg}}{50 \text{ mg / tablets}}$$

tablets required = 27 tablets

Step 2:
Since a loss of product may occur when preparing 90 doses, using 28 tablets will ensure that all doses can be obtained. Excess can be discarded or formulated into additional doses for later use. To determine the number of doses that we can theoretically be prepared from 28 tablets:

$$\text{doses available} = \frac{\text{strength of the tablet (mg)} \times \text{\# of tablets}}{\dfrac{\text{\# of mg}}{1 \text{ dose}}}$$

$$\text{doses available} = \frac{\dfrac{50 \text{ mg}}{1 \text{ tablet}} \times \dfrac{28 \text{ tablets}}{1}}{\dfrac{15 \text{ mg}}{1 \text{ dose}}}$$

$$\text{doses available} = \frac{1{,}400 \text{ mg}}{15 \text{ mg} / \text{dose}}$$

doses available = 93.3 doses

Step 3:
Weighing the 28 tablets on a Class I balance, you find that they weigh 4.21 g. Divide the weight of the tablets by the number of doses that can be prepared to calculate the weight of oxymethalone in each capsule:

$$\text{wt of each dose} = \frac{\text{wt of tablets}}{\text{\# of doses available}}$$

$$\text{wt of each dose} = \frac{4.21 \text{ g}}{93.3 \text{ doses}}$$

wt of each dose = 0.045 g

Step 4:
To convert from grams to milligrams, multiply by the factor 1000 mg per 1 g (See Appendix G):

$$\frac{0.045 \cancel{\text{ g}}}{1 \text{ dose}} \times \frac{1000 \text{ mg}}{1 \cancel{\text{ g}}} = 45 \text{ mg / dose}$$

The smallest empty gelatin capsule available is a #4, which you determine will hold 180 mg. To make up the difference between the 45 mg of drug and the 180 mg of space in the capsule, you will use a diluent such as lactose or milk sugar. To calculate the amount of diluent needed, multiply the number of doses possible (93.3) by 180 mg/dose and subtract the combined weight of the 28 tablets (4.21 g). Don't forget to use common units!

diluent required = (# of doses × wt of each dose) – wt of tablets

$$\text{diluent required} = 93.3 \text{ doses} \times \left(\frac{180 \cancel{\text{mg}}}{1 \text{ dose}} \times \frac{1 \text{ g}}{1000 \cancel{\text{mg}}} \right) - 4.21 \text{ g}$$

diluent required = (93.3 doses × 0.180 g/dose) – 4.21 g

diluent required = 16.794 – 4.21

diluent required = 12.584 g

Step 5:
Crush the tablets with a pestle in a mortar until it is a fine powder and add the 12.53 g of diluent (lactose) by geometric dilution (the volume added at any one time is approximately equal to that which it is being added to).

Step 6:
Pack each capsule to contain **180 mg (0.18 g)**. Don't forget to account for the weight of the empty gelatin capsule by placing the same size empty gelatin capsule on the opposite side of the balance!

★ **Example:** *Piroxicam (Feldene®) is suggested for the relief of pain associated with bladder cancer in a 34 lb dog at a dose of 5 mg every 24 hours. To make a 4 week supply,*

Step 1:
Determine the number of 10 mg capsules needed:

$$\text{total mg} = \frac{\text{mg}}{1 \text{ dose}} \times \frac{\text{\# of doses}}{1 \text{ day}} \times \frac{\text{\# of days}}{1}$$

$$\text{total mg} = \frac{5 \text{ mg}}{1 \text{ dose}} \times \frac{1 \text{ dose}}{1 \text{ day}} \times \frac{28 \text{ days}}{1}$$

total mg = 140 mg

Step 2:

$$\text{capsules needed} = \frac{\text{total number of mg required}}{\text{mg / commercial capsule}}$$

$$\text{capsules needed} = \frac{140 \text{ mg}}{10 \text{ mg / capsule}}$$

capsules needed = 14 capsules

Step 3:

Weigh out the contents of the 14 capsules.

If the contents of the 14 capsules weigh 3.78 g, how much will each dose weigh?

$$\frac{\text{single dose AI}}{\text{total doses AI}} = \frac{\text{wt of single dose}}{\text{wt of total doses}}$$

$$\frac{5 \text{ mg / dose}}{140 \text{ mg}} = \frac{\text{wt of single dose}}{3.78 \text{ g}}$$

Convert to common units and then solve the equation (See Appendix G):

$$\frac{3.78 \text{ g}}{1} \times \frac{1000 \text{ mg}}{1 \text{ g}} = 3780 \text{ mg}$$

$$\frac{5 \text{ mg / dose}}{140 \text{ mg}} = \frac{\text{single dose}}{3,780}$$

$$\text{single dose} \times 140 = 5 \times 3,780$$

$$\text{single dose} = \frac{5 \times 3,780}{140}$$

$$\text{single dose} = 135 \text{ mg per dose}$$

Step 4:

Each dose will weigh 135 mg, but the smallest capsule you have is a #4 and your technician can pack a #4 capsule to hold 190 mg of piroxicam. How much lactose should be added to make each capsule weigh 190 mg?

Determine the total mg of piroxicam required by using the formula:

$$\text{total mg required} = \frac{\text{mg}}{1 \text{ dose}} \times \frac{\text{\# of doses}}{1 \text{ day}} \times \frac{\text{\# of days}}{1}$$

$$\text{total mg required} = \frac{5 \text{ mg}}{1 \text{ dose}} \times \frac{1 \text{ dose}}{1 \text{ day}} \times \frac{28 \text{ days}}{1}$$

total mg required = 140 mg

Step 5:
Determine the number of doses that can be made from the 140 mg by dividing the number of milligrams per dose:

$$\frac{140 \text{ mg}}{5 \text{ mg / dose}} = 28 \text{ doses}$$

Step 6:
Multiply the 28 doses by 190 mg per dose to determine the total weight to be measured:

$$\text{total mg} = \frac{28 \text{ doses}}{1} \times \frac{190 \text{ mg}}{1 \text{ dose}}$$

$$\text{total g} = \frac{28}{1} \times \frac{190 \text{ mg}}{1} \times \frac{1 \text{ g}}{1000 \text{ mg}}$$

total g = 5.32 g

Step 7:
Subtract the weight of the 28 tablets from the total weight to determine the amount of lactose that should be added:

weight of lactose = total weight – weight of drug

weight of lactose = 5.32 g – 3.78 g piroxicam

weight of lactose = **1.54 g**

Alternative Method to Steps 1–7:

These calculations can be combined into a single step as illustrated below:

$$\text{diluent required} = \left(\frac{\text{total amount of AI}}{\text{amount of AI per dose}} \times \text{wt per dose} \right) - \text{wt of AI}$$

$$\text{diluent required} = \left(\frac{140 \ \cancel{mg} \ \text{total}}{5 \ \cancel{mg/dose}} \times 0.19 \ \text{g/}\cancel{dose} \right) - 3.78 \ \text{g}$$

diluent required = **1.54 g lactose**

Step 8:

Weigh out 1.54 g of the lactose and mix it with the contents of the 14 capsules then pack the mixture into #4 capsules each containing 190 mg. Don't forget to account for the weight of the empty gelatin capsule by placing one of the same size on the opposite pan of the balance.

Practice Problems
(See Appendix H for answers)

119. Lysodren® (Mitotane) is used to treat Cushing's disease at a dose of 23 mg/lb orally twice a week after an induction dose of 23 mg/lb daily for four to seven days. a) Determine the daily dose of mitotane needed to treat a 14 lb dog. b) Determine the number of 500 mg tablets of mitotane needed to treat this animal for 1 month at a dose of 23 mg/lb twice a week. c) Determine the amount of lactose needed if each tablet weighs 680 mg and each dose will be packed in a #1 capsule that holds 455 mg.

120. Oxazepam is sometimes used as an appetite stimulant in cats at a dose of 1.3 mg. Oxazepam is commercially available as 10, 15, and 30 mg capsules and 15 mg tablets. a) How many of the 10 mg capsules will be needed to make a 10 day supply if the cat is dosed once a day? b) If the contents of each oxazepam capsule weighs 140 mg, how much lactose should be added so that each #4 capsule weighs 180 mg?

121. DES (diethylstilbestrol) is occasionally used to treat urinary incontinence in cats at a dose of 0.05–0.1 mg once a day. The smallest commercially available tablet is 1 mg. a) How many tablets will be needed to treat a cat for 30 days at a dose of 0.1 mg? b) If 10 tablets weigh 800 mg, how much lactose is needed so that each #4 capsule weighs 180 mg?

122. Naltrexone has been used at a dose of 1–2 mg/kg orally daily for self-mutilation in dogs. a) How many of the 50 mg tablets would be needed to treat a 34 lb dog for 14 days at a dose of 1 mg/kg? b) To formulate each dose in a #3 capsule, how much lactose will be required if each tablet weighs 130 mg and the #3 capsule holds approximately 260 mg?

Oral Suspensions

★ **Example 1**: *Metronidazole is used to treat anaerobes in dogs and cats at a dose of 10–15 mg/kg orally every 8 hours. If you wish to treat a 6 lb cat for 5 days, how many of the 250 mg tablets would be needed to make a sufficient quantity of suspension?*

Step 1:
Establish common units by converting the weight of the cat from pounds to kilograms by multiplying by the factor 2.2 pounds equals 1 kilogram (See Appendix G):

$$\frac{6 \text{ lb}}{1} \times \frac{1 \text{ kg}}{2.2 \text{ lb}} = 2.7 \text{ kg}$$

Step 2:
To determine the amount of metronidazole required per dose, multiply the weight of the cat in kilograms by the dose of 10 mg/kg:

$$\frac{10 \text{ mg}}{\text{kg} / \text{dose}} \times \frac{2.7 \text{ kg}}{1} = 27 \text{ mg} / \text{dose}$$

Step 3:
Multiply the number of milligrams required per dose by the number of doses per day to determine the milligrams required per day:

$$\frac{27 \text{ mg}}{1 \text{ dose}} \times \frac{3 \text{ doses}}{1 \text{ day}} = 81 \text{ mg} / \text{day}$$

Step 4:
The result can be multiplied by the number of days to determine the total amount of metronidazole required:

$$\text{total mg} = \frac{27 \text{ mg}}{1 \text{ dose}} \times \frac{3 \text{ doses}}{\text{day}} \times \frac{5 \text{ days}}{1}$$

$$\text{total mg} = \frac{81 \text{ mg}}{1 \text{ day}} \times \frac{5 \text{ days}}{1}$$

$$\text{total mg} = 405 \text{ mg}$$

Step 5:
To determine the number of tablets required to provide 5 days of therapy for one 6 lb cat, divide the total amount of metronidazole required for 5 days of therapy (409 mg) by the strength of the commercial preparation (250 mg/tablet).

$$\text{\# of tablets } = \frac{405 \text{ mg}}{\dfrac{250 \text{ mg}}{1 \text{ tablet}}}$$

$$\text{\# of tablets } = \frac{405 \text{ mg}}{1} \times \frac{1 \text{ tablet}}{250 \text{ mg}}$$

# of tablets = 1.62 tablets ≈ 2 tablets

Step 6:
A 50 mg/ml suspension can be made by crushing the 2 tablets, placing the powder in a bottle, and adding equal volumes of water and corn syrup.

To determine the total volume required, multiply the number of the tablets (2) by their strength (250 mg/tablet) and divide by the desired concentration of the suspension (50 mg/ml).

$$\text{total volume required} = \frac{\text{total mg required}}{\text{concentration per ml}}$$

$$\text{total volume required} = \frac{\dfrac{2 \text{ tablets}}{1} \times \dfrac{250 \text{ mg}}{1 \text{ tablet}}}{50 \text{ mg / ml}}$$

$$\text{total volume required} = \frac{500 \text{ mg}}{50 \text{ mg / ml}}$$

total volume required = 10 ml

Compounding

Step 7:

Since corn syrup and water can be used in equal volumes, each will comprise 50% of the solution:

$$\frac{50\% \times 10\ ml}{100\%} = 5\ ml\ of\ each$$

Mix all ingredients together, shake well, and refrigerate. The resulting solution can be used for 30 days. The volume required to deliver each dose of 27 mg can be determined by setting up a ratio:

$$\frac{dose\ desired}{volume\ required} = \frac{concentration}{1\ ml}$$

Substituting the concentration of 50 mg/1 ml and the dose desired (27 mg) into this equation, we can determine the volume required to deliver the desired dose:

$$\frac{27\ mg}{volume\ required} = \frac{50\ mg}{1\ ml}$$

Cross multiply to solve the equation:

volume required × 50 = 27 × 1

volume required = **0.54 ml**

★ **Example:** *Dichlorphenamide (Daranide®) is used in the treatment of glaucoma. A dose of 10 mg per day is prescribed for a 20 lb dog to help control intraocular pressure. Daranide® is commercially available as 50 mg tablets. To make a 30 day supply:*

Step 1:

Calculate the number of tablets required:

$$\text{total mg required} = \frac{\text{mg}}{\text{dose}} \times \frac{\text{\# of doses}}{1 \text{ day}} \times \frac{\text{\# of days}}{1}$$

$$\text{total mg required} = \frac{10 \text{ mg}}{1} \times \frac{30}{1}$$

total mg required = 300 mg

Step 2:
Divide the total number of milligrams required by the strength of the tablets in milligrams to determine the number of tablets required:

$$\text{tablets required} = \frac{\text{mg required}}{\text{strength of one tablet}}$$

$$\text{tablets required} = \frac{300 \text{ mg}}{50 \text{ mg / tablet}}$$

tablets required = 6 tablets

Step 3:
Crush the tablets in a mortar to a fine powder. Place the powder in a 2 oz empty bottle. To recover all of the powder from the mortar and pestle, rinse them both with distilled or deionized water. Each will be rinsed with two aliquots of 5 ml each. Add 5 ml more of distilled or deionized water. Shake the dichlorphenamide and 15 ml of water well.

Step 4:
To determine the additional volume that is needed, you must first decide what volume you wish each dose to be delivered in. The volume of each dose should be sufficient to make it easy for the client to draw and administer, but not so much as to cause extreme stress to the patient. If the required dose to be delivered is

1 ml, first determine the total volume required. This is done by dividing the total number of milligrams required by the concentration desired per milliliter:

$$\text{total volume required} = \frac{\text{total mg required}}{\text{concentration per ml}}$$

$$\text{total volume required} = \frac{\dfrac{10 \text{ mg}}{1 \text{ day}} \times \dfrac{30 \text{ days}}{1}}{\dfrac{10 \text{ mg}}{1 \text{ ml}}}$$

$$\text{total volume required} = \frac{300 \text{ mg}}{10 \text{ mg} / \text{ml}}$$

total volume required = 30 ml

Step 5:
Thirty milliliters is the total volume required. To determine the amount of corn syrup and water that still needs to be added, subtract the volume of water that was used to rinse the mortar and pestle (15 ml) from the total volume required (30 ml):

30 ml – (5 ml + 5 ml + 5 ml) = 15 ml

Add 15 ml of corn syrup and shake well. Label: "Shake well and give 1 ml orally daily with food." The final concentration is 10 mg/ml.

Practice Problems
(See Appendix H for answers)

123. How many 250 mg tablets of metronidazole will be required to prepare 100 ml of a 25 mg/ml oral suspension?

124. If enrofloxacin is to be used to treat *Pseudomonas aeruginosa* at a dose of 7.5 mg/kg orally every 12 hours in a 3 lb puppy that the client can not pill, how many of the 68 mg tablets should be crushed and made into a suspension to provide 10 days of therapy?

125. If 20 mg/kg/day of ketoconazole is needed to treat a 90 g cockatiel, in how many milliliters of pineapple juice should one 200 mg tablet be dissolved to provide each dose in 0.1 ml?

Eye Drops

★ **Example:** *Cyclosporine has been found to be useful in increasing tear production in animals affected with KCS. A 2% cyclosporine eye drop can be made using the oral 10% preparation. Calculate the amount of 10% cyclosporine solution needed to make 5 ml of the 2% eye drops by setting up an equation:*

volume × strength = volume × strength

Place the desired product (volume and strength) on one side and the volume and strength of the stock solution on the other. In this case we are solving for the volume of the stock solution:

5 ml × 2% = unknown volume (ml) × 10%

$$\text{unknown volume} = \frac{5 \text{ ml} \times 2\%}{10\%}$$

unknown volume = **1 ml**

Add 1 ml of the commercial 10% solution to 4 ml of extra virgin olive oil and filter sterilize through a 0.22 micrometer filter into a sterile 7 ml dropper bottle. The resulting solution is stable for 60 days at room temperature.

★ **Example:** *Sodium penicillin has been used to treat Beta Streptococcus eye infections by making a solution of artificial tears containing 166,667 U/ml. If you have a 5 million unit vial, how much artificial tears is needed to make a 166,667 U/ml solution?*

Step 1:
Determine the number of ml of 166,667 U/ml that can be made from the 5 million unit vial.

$$\text{ml / vial} = \frac{\text{concentration / vial}}{\text{desired concentration / ml}}$$

$$\text{ml / vial} = \frac{5{,}000{,}000 \text{ U / vial}}{166{,}667 \text{ U / ml}}$$

ml/vial = 29.999 ml ≈ **30 ml**

Step 2:
Reconstitute the 5,000,000 unit vial with 4.5 ml sterile water for injection. The resulting solution will be 1,000,000 U/ml. Mix well and let stand until the penicillin dissolves and a solution is formed. To determine the amount of artificial tears needed, subtract the volume occupied by the sodium penicillin from the total volume that can be made. Since the volume to be occupied by sodium penicillin is 5 ml, subtract this amount from the total volume calculated to determine the amount of artificial tears needed:

total volume = volume of medicine + diluent

total volume = volume of sodium penicillin + volume of artificial tears

30 ml = 5 ml + volume of artificial tears

volume of artificial tears = **25 ml**

Draw up the contents of vial (5 ml) and add 25 ml of artificial tears to make a final volume of 30 ml. The resulting solution is stable for one week under refrigeration.

Practice Problems
(See Appendix H for answers)

126. To make a fortified gentamicin ophthalmic solution of 10 mg/ml, how much of the 50 mg/ml injectable preparation should be added to 5 ml of Gentocin® (3 mg/ml gentamicin)? (Hint: The final volume will be more than 5 ml).

127. If 1.7 ml of 50 mg/ml gentamicin is added to 5 ml of Gentocin® ophthalmic solution, what is the final concentration?

128. If 3 g of disodium edetate, 300 mg of sodium chloride, and 0.058 ml of Zephiran® 17% solution are combined in 100 ml of water for injection and filter sterilized to make disodium EDTA ophthalmic drops, what is the final concentration of disodium edetate?

129. To make a 100 mg/ml cephaperin ophthalmic solution, how many milliliters of artificial tears should be used to reconstitute a 1 gram vial of cephaperin?

130. If 0.6 ml of Synacid® is added to Adapt® for a final volume of 15 ml and a final concentration of 0.04% Synacid®, what is the original strength of Synacid®?

Topical Preparations

★ **Example:** *Tris-EDTA solution is sometimes used to treat pseudomonal infections on the skin and in the ears. Gentamicin, amikacin, or oxytetracycline is sometimes added to increase its efficacy. You wish to make a Tris-EDTA solution containing gentamicin. How much gentamicin is needed to make 2 oz of a 3 mg/ml preparation?*

Step 1:
Convert to common units (See Appendix G):

1 oz = 29.57 ml ≈ 30 ml
2 oz × (30 ml/oz) = 60 ml

Step 2:
To determine the amount of gentamicin required, multiply the final concentration of gentamicin desired by the final volume desired:

amount required = final concentration × final volume

$$\text{drug required} = \frac{60 \ \cancel{ml}}{1} \times \frac{3 \ mg}{1 \ \cancel{ml}}$$

drug required = 180 mg

Step 3:
Gentamicin is available as a 50 mg/ml preparation. To determine the number of milliliters of the 50 mg/ml preparation needed to provide the 180 mg, divide the

number of milligrams required by the concentration of the commercial preparation in mg per ml:

$$\text{ml of commercial prep} = \frac{\text{\# of mg required}}{\text{conc commercial prep (mg / ml)}}$$

$$\text{ml of commercial prep} = \frac{180 \text{ mg}}{\dfrac{50 \text{ mg}}{1 \text{ ml}}}$$

$$\text{ml of commercial prep} = \frac{180 \text{ mg}}{50 \text{ mg / ml}}$$

ml of commercial prep = **3.6 ml**

Add 3.6 ml of 50 mg/ml gentamicin to 56.4 ml of Tris-EDTA.

★ **Example:** *Furacin-glycerin sweat is made by mixing equal volumes of glycerin and nitrofurazone solution. If furacin-glycerin sweat is to be applied to a horse's leg at each bandage change, how many pints of furacin-glycerin sweat can be made using 1 gallon of nitrofurazone?*

Convert to common units (See Appendix G):

2 pints = 1 quart
4 quarts = 1 gallon

Because nitrofurazone comprises only 50% of the concentration, 2 gallons can be made using 1 gallon of nitrofurazone. By inserting the above conversions from gallons to quarts to pints, it can be determined how many pints of furacin-glycerin sweat can be made.

$$\frac{2\ \text{gal}}{1} \times \frac{4\ \text{qt}}{1\ \text{gal}} \times \frac{2\ \text{pt}}{1\ \text{qt}} = 16\ \text{pints}$$

Practice Problems
(See Appendix H for answers)

131. Hot spot cocktail can be made using 60 ml of dimethyl sulfoxide gel, 30 ml of 2 mg/ml dexamethasone, and 12 ml of flunixin 50 mg/ml injection and adding distilled or deionized water to a total volume of 120 ml. a) What is the final concentration of dexamethasone in mg/ml? b) What is final concentration of flunixin in mg/ml? c) What percentage of the preparation is represented by dimethyl sulfoxide?

132. How much iodine is needed to make 1 pint of strong iodine (7%)?

133. VUT #3 (Volume Uterine Treatment) is infused into the uterus every other day at a dose of 50 ml. To make 4,000 ml, how much nitrofurazone 0.2% solution is used if the final concentration of nitrofurazone is 0.1265%?

134. What is the final percentage of oxytetracycline if 20 g of oxytetracycline powder are contained in 4,000 ml of solution?

135. Modified Dankin's solution can be prepared using 47.5 ml of bleach (5.25% sodium hypochlorite), 1.2 ml of 8.4% sodium bicarbonate injection, and adding water to a total volume of 500 ml. a) What is the final percentage of sodium hypochlorite if its initial concentration is 5.25%? b) What is the final concentration of sodium bicarbonate in mcg/ml?

Nutritional Support

Determining Nutritional Needs

Nutritional support can be provided enterally using the alimentary canal or parenterally (intravenously). If an animal will not eat, nutrition can be provided enterally via a nasogastric tube, gastric tube, duodenal tube, or jejunostomy tube. If the gastrointestinal tract is working, it should be utilized because 1) nutrients can be provided less expensively, 2) the gastrointestinal tract acts like a filter, absorbing through passive and facilitated transport those nutrients that the body needs and not absorbing entities that are not required or that could be harmful, and 3) if the cells of the gastrointestinal tract are not fed, they begin to die, allowing uncontrolled movement of elements into and out of the body. If the gastrointestinal tract cannot be utilized or all of the nutritional needs cannot be met enterally, parenteral nutrition should be considered.

Parenteral nutrition can be provided by peripheral or central access. Central access is obtained through a large vein (e.g., external jugular). Central access allows very concentrated solutions to be administered. These solutions are hypertonic (1000 + mOsm) and would cause phlebitis, irritation, and pain if given in a peripheral vein.

Peripheral access is through any small vein in the leg or wing. Solutions may be slightly hypertonic (up to 500–600 mOsm) such as a 10% dextrose solution or 5% dextrose with 2–3% amino acids. The primary reason that peripheral veins are not commonly used is the large volumes of solutions that are required to meet nutritional requirements.

Nutritional support requires the calculation of basal energy expenditure and adjusted energy expenditure. When nutritional support is provided via J-tube,

NG tube, PEG tube, or parenterally the rate and composition of the nutrients must be calculated.

Summary Formulas

I. Basal Energy Requirements (BER):
   a) Mammals: $70 \times$ (wt in kg)$^{0.75}$
      e.g., dog, cat, cow, horse
   b) Marsupials: $49 \times$ (wt in kg)$^{0.75}$
      e.g., opossum, wallabies, kangaroos
   c) Passerine birds: $129 \times$ (wt in kg)$^{0.75}$
      e.g., songbirds, pigeons, doves
   d) Nonpasserine birds: $78 \times$ (wt in kg)$^{0.75}$
      e.g., raptors, geese, psittacines
   e) Reptiles: $10 \times$ (wt in kg)$^{0.75}$
      e.g., snakes, turtles, lizards

II. Adjusted Energy Requirements (AER):
   a) Enclosure rest: 1 to $1.25 \times$ BER
   b) Starvation: 1 to $1.25 \times$ BER
   c) Postsurgery: $1.25 \times$ BER
   d) Severe burns: 1.5 to $2 \times$ BER
   e) Sepsis: 1.5 to $2 \times$ BER
   f) Trauma: $1.5 \times$ BER
   g) Cancer: $1.5 \times$ BER
   h) Hepatic disease: $1.25 \times$ BER
   i) Severe renal disease (e.g., BUN > 80): $1.25 \times$ BER

III. Grams of nitrogen = AER/Kcal / gram of nitrogen for I.V. administration

IV. Daily feed requirement $= \dfrac{\text{Kcal required / day}}{\text{caloric content of the diet}}$

total nonprotein calories =
Kcal provided by lipids + Kcal provided by dextrose

quantity of dextrose solution required =

$$\frac{\text{Kcal of dextrose needed}}{\text{conc of dextrose (Kcal / ml)}}$$

$$\text{g of nitrogen required} = \frac{\text{total calories}}{\text{Kcal to N ratio}}$$

$$\text{g of amino acids} = \text{g of nitrogen} \times \frac{6.25 \text{ g amino acids}}{1 \text{ g N}}$$

quantity of amino acid solution required =

$$\frac{\text{g of AA needed}}{\text{conc of AA solution (g / 100 ml)}}$$

volume of additives =
total volume − (volume for calories + volume of proteins)

Note: Food calories are referred to as kilocalories (Kcal). Kilocalories are used when determining caloric requirements.

Metabolic Scaling

Basal Energy Requirements (BER)
The basal metabolic rate is the minimal amount of energy required to maintain body function in an animal. Energy requirements are modified by stage of life, environmental conditions, and disease. Maintenance energy requirements (MER) for animals are usually 1.5 to 2 times the basal energy requirement (BER) and under some conditions energy requirements may be 3 times the basal energy requirement. As listed earlier, basal energy requirements may be calculated using the equations:

a) Mammals: $70 \times$ (wt in kg)$^{0.75}$

  e.g., dog, cat, cow, horse

b) Marsupials: $49 \times$ (wt in kg)$^{0.75}$

  e.g., opossum, wallabies, kangaroos

c) Passerine birds: $129 \times$ (wt in kg)$^{0.75}$

  e.g., songbirds, pigeons, doves

d) Nonpasserine birds: $78 \times$ (wt in kg)$^{0.75}$

  e.g., raptors, geese, psittacines

e) Reptiles: $10 \times$ (wt in kg)$^{0.75}$

  e.g., snakes, turtles, lizards

★ **Example:** *To determine the BER of a 10 lb cat, convert the animal's weight from pounds to kilograms (See Appendix G):*

Step 1:

$$\frac{\text{wt (lb)}}{1} \times \frac{1 \text{ kg}}{2.2 \text{ lb}} = \text{kg}$$

$$\frac{10 \text{ lb}}{1} \times \frac{1 \text{ kg}}{2.2 \text{ lb}} = 4.5 \text{ kg}$$

Step 2:

Then insert the weight in kilograms into the equation for mammals: BER = $70 \times$ (wt in kg)$^{0.75}$

BER = $70 \times (4.5)^{0.75}$

BER = 70×3.09

BER = **216 Kcal/day**

Note: *If you do not have a y^x key on your calculator, find $y^{0.75}$ by first multiplying $y \times y \times y$. (See Appendix J.) Then, take the square root of the product. Finally, take the square root again. For example:*

$4.5 \times 4.5 \times 4.5 = 91.125$

$\sqrt{91.125} = 9.545$

$\sqrt{9.545} = 3.09$

★ **Example:** *To determine the BER for a 10 lb kangaroo, convert the animal's weight from pounds to kilograms:*

$$\frac{\text{wt (lb)}}{1} \times \frac{1 \text{ kg}}{2.2} = \text{kg}$$

$$\frac{10 \cancel{\text{lb}}}{1} \times \frac{1 \text{ kg}}{2.2 \cancel{\text{lb}}} = 4.5 \text{ kg}$$

Then insert the weight of the animal in kilograms into the equation for marsupials:

$\text{BER} = 49 \times (\text{wt in kg})^{0.75}$

$\text{BER} = 49 \times (4.5)^{0.75}$

$\text{BER} = 49 \times 3.09$

$\text{BER} = \textbf{151 Kcal/day}$

★ **Example:** *To determine the BER for a 45 g bluebird, convert the animal's weight from grams to kilograms:*

$$\frac{\text{wt (g)}}{1} \times \frac{1 \text{ kg}}{1000 \text{ g}} = \text{kg}$$

$$\frac{45 \cancel{\text{g}}}{1} \times \frac{1 \text{ kg}}{1000 \cancel{\text{g}}} = 0.045 \text{ kg}$$

Then insert the weight in kilograms into the equation for passerines:

$$BER = 129 \times (wt \ in \ kg)^{0.75}$$

$$BER = 129 \times (0.045)^{0.75}$$

$$BER = 129 \times 0.0977$$

$$BER = \textbf{12.6 Kcal/day}$$

★ **Example:** *To determine the BER for a 3 lb 2 oz redtail hawk, convert the animal's weight from ounces and pounds to pounds using the conversion factor 16 oz = 1 lb.*

$$\frac{3 \ lb}{1} + \left(\frac{2 \ \cancel{oz}}{1} \times \frac{1 \ lb}{16 \ \cancel{oz}} \right) = 3.125 \ lb$$

Then convert the weight to kilograms using the conversion factor 2.2 lb = 1 kg

$$\frac{3.125 \ \cancel{lb}}{1} \times \frac{1 \ kg}{2.2 \ \cancel{lb}} = 1.42 \ kg$$

and insert the weight in kilograms into the equation for nonpasserines:

$$BER = 78 \times (wt \ in \ kg)^{0.75}$$

$$BER = 78 \times (1.42)^{0.75}$$

$$BER = 78 \times 1.3$$

$$BER = \textbf{101.4 Kcal/day}$$

★ **Example:** *To determine the BER for a 7 lb boa constrictor, convert the animal's weight to kilograms:*

$$\frac{7 \ \cancel{lb}}{1} \times \frac{1 \ kg}{2.2 \ \cancel{lb}} = 3.18 \ kg$$

and insert the weight in kilograms into the equation for
BER = $10 \times$ (wt in kg)$^{0.75}$

BER = $10 \times (3.18)^{0.75}$

BER = 10×2.38

BER = **23.8 Kcal/day**

Practice Problems
(See Appendix H for answers)

136. Determine the BER for a 90 lb dog.
137. Determine the BER for a 12 lb opossum.
138. Determine the BER for a 1 kg dove.
139. Determine the BER for a 10 kg goose.
140. Determine the BER for a 42 lb turtle.

Adjusted Energy Requirements (AER)

After calculating the basal energy requirement, the
amount of energy to be provided should be adjusted to
include the increased need for energy created by disease or injury by multiplying the basal energy requirement (BER) by the factor of the appropriate disease
state repeated below. The result is the adjusted energy
requirement (AER).

    a) Enclosure rest: 1 to $1.25 \times$ BER
    b) Starvation: 1 to $1.25 \times$ BER
    c) Postsurgery: $1.25 \times$ BER
    d) Severe burns: 1.5 to $2 \times$ BER
    e) Sepsis: 1.5 to $2 \times$ BER
    f) Trauma: $1.5 \times$ BER
    g) Cancer: $1.5 \times$ BER
    h) Hepatic disease: $1.25 \times$ BER
    i) Severe renal disease (e.g., BUN > 80): $1.25 \times$
       BER

Note: If multiple disease states exist, use the value for the disease state that has the highest AER unless renal disease is present. If renal disease is present, use i).

Caloric requirements are also increased in growth, gestation, and lactation. Energy requirements during periods of growth are approximately 1.5 to 2 times the BER.

★ **Example:** *You evaluate an 18-year-old 7 lb cat with renal disease. It is not eating and you decide to begin feedings with Feline Renal Care®. What is this cat's a) BER, b) AER, c) and how much Feline Renal Care® does it need each day?*

a) To estimate the BER for this cat, use the equation for mammals:

$$BER = 70 \times (wt \; in \; kg)^{0.75}$$

Convert the weight from pounds to kilograms using the conversion factor of 2.2 pounds per kilograms (See Appendix G).

$$\frac{7 \; \cancel{lb}}{1} \times \frac{1 \; kg}{2.2 \; \cancel{lb}} = 3.18 \; kg$$

Then insert the weight in kilograms in the above equation:

$$BER = 70 \times (3.18)^{0.75}$$

If you do not have a calculator with a y^x key, refer to Appendix J.

$$BER = 70 \times 2.38 = 166.6 \; Kcal/day$$

If the weight was rounded to 3 kg, a value of 2.28 would be used and inserted into the equation instead of the calculated 2.38. The resulting BER would be 159.6 or **160 Kcal per day.**

b) Energy requirements should be adjusted based on disease state. Since this cat is in severe renal disease, the AER equation for severe renal disease should be used; that is, severe renal disease (BUN > 80): AER = 125 × BER.

AER = (conversion factor for disease) × BER
AER = 1.25 × BER
AER = 1.25 × 166.8 Kcal/day
AER = **213.5 Kcal/day**

c) To determine the amount of Feline Renal Care® that should be fed each day, divide the number of Kcal required by the caloric content of the nutritional supplement. Feline Renal Care® contains 0.84 Kcal/ml.

$$\text{daily feed requirement} = \frac{\text{Kcal required / day}}{\text{caloric content of diet}}$$

$$\text{feed requirement} = \frac{213.5 \text{ Kcal/day}}{0.84 \text{ Kcal/ml}}$$

feed requirement = **254 ml/day**

The 254 ml of Feline Renal Care® should be divided into 4 to 6 feedings per day. While Feline Renal Care® is iso-osmotic, many practitioners find it useful to dilute enteral feedings with an equal volume of water for the first 24 hours to minimize diarrhea and vomiting.

★ **Example:** *An 8-month-old, 47 lb dog is referred to your clinic to rule out obstruction. Exploratory surgery is performed and the gear shift handle from the client's car is removed. You wish to initiate enteral feeding and place a gastrostomy tube. You have K9 Clinicare® in the pharmacy. What is this dog's a) BER, b) AER, c) and how much K9 Clinicare® does the patient need each day?*

a) To estimate the BER, use the equation for mammals:

$$BER = 70 \times (wt\ in\ kg)^{0.75}$$

Convert the weight from pounds to kilograms using the conversion factor 2.2 lb = 1 kg (See Appendix G).

$$\frac{47\ \cancel{lb}}{1} \times \frac{1\ kg}{2.2\ \cancel{lb}} = 21.4\ kg$$

Then insert the weight in kilograms in the above equation:

$$BER = 70 \times (21.4)^{0.75}$$

If you do not have a calculator with a y^x key, refer to Appendix J.

$$BER = 70 \times 9.94 = \textbf{696 Kcal/day}$$

b) Energy requirements should be adjusted based on the disease state in this case:

Enclosure rest: 1 to 1.25 × BER
Postsurgery: 1.25 × BER

If multiple disease states are present, the factor for the disease state with the largest value should be used. This patient is postsurgical and will be resting in a restricted enclosure, so the adjusted energy requirement is

AER = 1.25 × BER
AER = 1.25 × 696
AER = **870 Kcal/day.**

c) To determine the amount of K9 Clinicare® that should be fed each day, divide the number of Kcal required by the caloric content of the nutritional supplement. K9 Clinicare® contains 0.98 Kcal/ml.

$$\text{daily feed requirement} = \frac{\text{Kcal required / day}}{\text{caloric content of the diet}}$$

$$\text{feed requirement} = \frac{870 \text{ Kcal / day}}{0.98 \text{ Kcal / ml}}$$

feed requirement = **888 ml/day**

The 888 ml should be divided into 4 to 6 feedings per day. While K9 Clinicare® is iso-osmotic, many practitioners find it useful to dilute enteral feedings with an equal volume of water for the first 24 hours to minimize diarrhea and vomiting.

★ **Example:** *A 10 kg wallaby is refusing to eat after the loss of her mate 10 days ago. You decide to provide enteral nutritional support. a) Estimate the BER, b) AER, and c) volume of the nutritional supplement required each day.*

a) To estimate the BER, use the equation for marsupials.

BER = 49 × (wt in kg)$^{0.75}$

Then insert the weight in kilograms in the above equation:

BER = 49 × (10)$^{0.75}$

If you do not have a calculator with a y^x key, refer to Appendix J.

BER = 49 × 5.62
BER = **275.38 Kcal/day**

b) Energy requirements should be adjusted based on the disease state in this case:

Starvation: 1 to 1.25 × BER

This animal has not eaten for 10 days and is losing weight, so the adjusted energy requirement for starvation is

AER = 1.25 × BER
AER = 1.25 × 275.5 Kcal/day
AER = **344.4 Kcal/day**

c) You decide to stomach tube the wallaby with Osmolite HN® obtained from your local hospital. Osmolite HN® is an isotonic, low residue, nutritional supplement providing approximately 1 Kcal/ml. To determine the amount of Osmolite HN® required per day, divide the adjusted energy requirement (AER) by the caloric content of the nutritional supplement:

$$\text{daily feed requirement} = \frac{\text{Kcal required / day}}{\text{caloric content of the diet}}$$

$$\text{daily feed requirement} = \frac{344.4 \text{ Kcal / day}}{1.06 \text{ Kcal / ml}}$$

daily feed requirement = 324.90 ≈ **325 ml/day**

You decide to stomach tube the wallaby six times a day for three days and decrease feedings as her appetite increases. You dilute the Osmolite HN® with an equal volume of water for the first 24 hours and feed the animal 50 ml a feeding. How many calories will the wallaby receive the first day?

$$\frac{50 \text{ ml}}{1 \text{ } \cancel{\text{feeding}}} \times \frac{6 \text{ } \cancel{\text{feeding}}}{1 \text{ day}} = \frac{300 \text{ ml}}{1 \text{ day}}$$

$$\frac{300 \text{ } \cancel{\text{ml}}}{1 \text{ day}} \times \frac{1 \text{ Kcal}}{1 \text{ } \cancel{\text{ml}}} = \frac{300 \text{ Kcal}}{1 \text{ day}}$$

The Osmolite has been diluted with an equal volume of water, so it only contains half as many calories:

$$\frac{1}{2} \times \frac{300 \text{ Kcal}}{1 \text{ day}} = 150 \text{ Kcal / day}$$

★ **Example:** *A 700 g blue and gold macaw chick is presented with a three day history of anorexia. Physical examination reveals emaciation, diarrhea, and 5–10% dehydration. An intraosseous catheter is placed in the ulna to deliver LRS, and Vital HN® is chosen to provide caloric support for the patient. Vital HN® is an elemental, partially hydrolyzed protein, low fat, low residue enteral supplement providing 1 Kcal/ml. To determine the amount of Vital HN® that should be provided, calculate a) the BER, b) the AER, and c) divide the AER by the caloric content of the nutritional supplement to determine the volume to be administered each day.*

a) To determine the BER, convert the animal's weight from grams to kilograms (See Appendix G):

$$\frac{700 \cancel{g}}{1} \times \frac{1 \text{ kg}}{1000 \cancel{g}} = 0.7 \text{ kg}$$

Then choose the equation for nonpasserine birds and insert the animal's weight in kilograms in the equation:

$$BER = 78 \times (0.7)^{0.75}$$

If you do not have a calculator with a y^x function key see Appendix J.

$$BER = 78 \times 0.765$$
$$BER = 59.7 \approx 60 \text{ Kcal/day}$$

b) The AER can be calculated by taking into account both disease state and stage of life. Energy requirements during periods of growth are approximately 1.5 to 2 times the BER. The requirements for growth exceed those of starvation and so this value is used.

$$AER = 1.5 \times BER$$
$$AER = 1.5 \times 60 \text{ Kcal/day}$$
$$AER = 90 \text{ Kcal/day}$$

c) To determine the amount of Vital HN® required, divide the daily caloric requirement by the caloric content of the nutritional supplement:

$$\text{daily feed requirement} = \frac{\text{Kcal required}}{\text{caloric content diet}}$$

$$\text{daily feed requirement} = \frac{\dfrac{90 \text{ Kcal}}{1 \text{ day}}}{\dfrac{1 \text{ Kcal}}{1 \text{ ml}}}$$

$$\text{daily feed requirement} = \frac{90 \text{ Kcal}}{1 \text{ day}} \times \frac{1 \text{ ml}}{1 \text{ Kcal}}$$

daily feed requirement = 90 ml/day

If the chick is to be fed four times a day, divide the volume to be fed by the number of feedings to determine the volume per feeding:

$$\text{volume / feeding} = \frac{\text{total volume}}{\text{\# of feedings}}$$

$$\text{volume/feeding} = \frac{90 \text{ ml}}{4}$$

volume/feeding = **22.5 ml/feeding**

★ **Example**: *A 2-week-old squirrel is presented with lethargy, anorexia, and dehydration. If the squirrel weighs 45 g and requires 150 Kcal/kg, how much of a 1 Kcal/ml oral replacement solution should it receive each day?*

Step 1:
Convert the weight from grams to kilograms (See Appendix G):

$$\frac{45 \cancel{g}}{1} \times \frac{1 \text{ kg}}{1000 \cancel{g}} = 0.045 \text{ kg}$$

Step 2:
Multiply the caloric requirement per kilogram by the weight in kilograms:

$$\frac{150 \text{ Kcal}}{1 \cancel{kg}} \times \frac{0.045 \cancel{kg}}{1} = 6.75 \text{ Kcal}$$

Step 3:

Divide the daily caloric requirement by the caloric content of the solution to determine the volume needed per day:

$$\text{volume / day} = \frac{\dfrac{6.75 \text{ Kcal}}{1 \text{ day}}}{\dfrac{1 \text{ Kcal}}{1 \text{ ml}}}$$

$$\text{volume / day} = \frac{6.75 \text{ \cancel{Kcal}}}{1 \text{ day}} \times \frac{1 \text{ ml}}{1 \text{ \cancel{Kcal}}}$$

volume/day = **6.75 ml/day**

Divide the 6.75 ml per day into 4 to 8 feedings. Warm the fluids to normal body temperature before administering. Never give food to a hypothermic animal. Fluids may be administered by a stomach tube if the animal is unresponsive.

Practice Problems
(See Appendix H for answers)

141. Determine the AER for a 10 kg black bear cub that has not eaten in three days.
142. Determine the AER for a 30 kg kangaroo that is septic.
143. Determine the AER for a 75 g goldfinch that has suffered a broken beak and wing after running into a window.
144. Determine the AER for a 20 kg goose that has just had surgery.
145. Determine the AER for a 5 kg iguana that has hepatic disease.

Parenteral Nutrition

Parenteral nutrition is a means of supplying the nutritional requirements of an animal when oral feeding is not feasible. Nutritional support may be provided by a central line or peripherally. Central lines utilize large, rapidly flowing veins (e.g., external jugular) that allow the administration of hypertonic solutions (1000 or more mOsm/L). The nutritional requirements of most patients can be adequately met even when fluid is restricted. This dedicated central line must be aseptically placed and used for nothing except providing nutritional support. To prevent contamination of the line, not even blood samples are to be taken from this line.

A peripheral line is usually in a smaller, slower flowing vein. The limiting factor in utilizing peripheral vessels is the osmolarity of the fluid that can be administered. Approximately two times iso-osmotic or the equivalent of 10% dextrose (or 5% dextrose + 3% amino acids) is the maximum osmolarity that can be administered through a peripheral line. Thus, larger volumes of nutritional products must be administered to meet the animal's nutritional requirements. Volumes required may exceed the fluid tolerance of the patient in some cases (e.g., renal disease). Peripheral lines are used for short-term nutritional support. The calculations of nutritional requirements are contained in the following section. This section is not meant to provide clinical information. Please refer to an appropriate text for information regarding TPN (total parenteral nutrition).

Nutritional Support Requirements	
a) Enclosure rest	1 g N: 125 to 150 Kcal
b) Nonstress starvation	1 g N: 125 to 150 Kcal
c) Postsurgery	1 g N: 125 Kcal
d) Severe burns	1 g N: 80 to 100 Kcal
e) Sepsis	1 g N: 80 to 125 Kcal
f) Trauma	1g N: 100 to 125 Kcal
g) Cancer	1 g N: 100 to 125 Kcal
h) Hepatic insufficiency	1 g N: 200 Kcal
i) Severe renal disease	1 g N: 200 to 500 Kcal

★ **Example 1:** *A 100 lb embryo transfer calf has developed diarrhea. You place it on the antibiotics ceftiofur and metronidazole. The diarrhea stops but the calf won't eat. Develop a TPN protocol for this calf. Start by calculating the basal energy requirement (BER).*

Step 1:
Convert the weight from pounds to kilograms (See Appendix G):

$$\frac{100 \text{ lb}}{1} \times \frac{1 \text{ kg}}{2.2 \text{ lb}} = 45.45 \text{ kg}$$

Insert the weight in kilograms into the BER equation for mammals. If you don't have a scientific calculator with a y^x function key, see Appendix J.

BER = $70 \times (45.45)^{0.75}$
BER = 70×17.5
BER = **1,225 Kcal/day**

You adjust the energy requirement for growth by multiplying the BER by a factor of 1.5. The adjusted energy requirement is

AER = BER × 1.5

AER = 1,225 Kcal/day × 1.5

AER = **1,838 Kcal**

Step 2:
To determine the amount of protein required, divide
the number of Kcal by the 1 g N: 150 Kcal ratio used
in growth:

$$\text{protein required} = \frac{1,838 \ \cancel{\text{Kcal}}}{1} \times \frac{1 \text{ g N}}{150 \ \cancel{\text{Kcal}}}$$

protein required = 12.25 g N

There are 6.25 g of amino acids (AA)/g N. Thus,

$$\text{AA required} = \frac{12.25 \ \cancel{\text{g N}}}{1} \times \frac{6.25 \text{ g AA}}{1 \ \cancel{\text{g N}}}$$

AA required = **76.56 g (AA)**

Step 3:
To determine the amount of a 10% amino acid (AA)
solution that will be needed, divide the amino acid
requirement by 10 g of amino acids per 100 ml:

$$\text{volume needed} = \frac{76.56 \text{ g AA}}{\dfrac{10 \text{ g AA}}{100 \text{ ml}}}$$

$$\text{volume needed} = \frac{76.56 \ \cancel{\text{g AA}}}{1} \times \frac{100 \text{ ml}}{10 \ \cancel{\text{g AA}}}$$

volume needed = 76.56 × 10 ml

volume needed = **766 ml**

Parenteral Nutrition Worksheet for Example 1

1. Basal Energy Requirements = __1,225__
   ✓Mammals: 70 × (wt in kg)$^{0.75}$
   Marsupials: 49 × (wt in kg)$^{0.75}$
   Passerine birds: 129 × (wt in kg)$^{0.75}$
   Nonpasserine birds: 78 × (wt in kg)$^{0.75}$
   Reptiles: 10 × (wt in kg)$^{0.75}$

2. Adjusted Energy Requirements = __1,838__
   Cage rest/Nonstress starvation: 1 to 1.25 × BER
   Postsurgery/Hepatic insufficiency: 1.25 × BER
   Severe renal disease: 1.25 × BER
   Trauma/Cancer: 1.5 × BER
   Burns/Sepsis: 1.75 to 2 × BER
   ✓Growth: 1.5 to 2 × BER

3. Protein Requirements = __12.25__ grams nitrogen

Cage rest	1 g N: 125 to150 Kcal
Nonstress starvation	1 g N: 125 to150 Kcal
Postsurgery	1 g N: 125 Kcal
Hepatic insufficiency	1 g N: 200 Kcal
Severe renal disease	1 g N: 200 to 500 Kcal
Trauma/Cancer	1 g N: 100 Kcal
Burns/Sepsis	1 g N: 80 to 100 Kcal
✓Growth	1 g N: 150 Kcal

4. Volume Requirements
   a) Protein: 10% AA __766__ ml   (6.25 g AA/1 g N)
      max. utilization: 3 g AA/kg/day   (810 mOsm/L)
   b) Lipids: 20% _____ ml   (2 Kcal/ml)
      max. utilization: 2.5 g/kg/day   (260 mOsm/L)
   c) Dextrose: 50% _____ ml   (1.7 Kcal/ml)
      optimal rate: 7–10 g/kg/day   (2,526 mOsml/L)

★ **Example 2:** *A 44 lb dog has been hit by a car. It has multiple broken bones, including a mandible that has to be surgically closed to facilitate healing. Develop a TPN treatment for this dog.*

Step 1:

Choose the BER equation for mammals.

BER for Mammals: 70 × (wt in kg)$^{0.75}$

Convert the weight from lb to kg.

$$\frac{44 \cancel{lb}}{1} \times \frac{1 \text{ kg}}{2.2 \cancel{lb}} = 20 \text{ kg}$$

Insert the weight and calculate the BER.

BER = 70 × (20)$^{0.75}$
BER = 70 × 9.46
BER = **662 Kcal/day**

Step 2:

The adjusted energy requirement must take into account both trauma and surgery. Since neither renal disease or hepatic insufficiency are involved, we should use the value for the disease state with the highest adjusted energy expenditure. The AER for surgery is 1.25 × BER; the AER for trauma is 1.5 × BER. Using the AER for trauma, we calculate the adjusted energy requirement to be

AER = 1.5 × BER
AER = 1.5 × 662
AER = **993 Kcal/day**

Step 3:

With trauma, the provided carbohydrates may not be fully utilized. Additionally, fluid restriction is indicated in injuries involving the head. Thus, you decide to provide 60% of the required nonprotein calories using lipids. Unless otherwise specified, a solution containing 20% lipids will be used in the calculations. (A 20% lipid solution provides 2 Kcal/ml).

Kcal from lipids = AER × percentage of calories from lipids

Kcal from lipids = 993 Kcal × 0.6

Kcal from lipids = 595.8 ≈ 596 Kcal

$$\text{ml of } 20\% \text{ lipids} = \frac{\text{Kcal from lipids}}{2 \text{ Kcal / ml of } 20\% \text{ lipids}}$$

$$\text{ml of lipids} = \frac{596 \text{ Kcal}}{2 \text{ Kcal / ml of } 20\% \text{ lipids}}$$

ml of lipids =298 ml ≈ 300 ml of 20% lipids ≈ **600 Kcal**

Step 4:
If 60% of nonprotein calories are coming from lipids, then 40% (100 – 60%) should be obtained in the form of dextrose. Unless otherwise specified, 50% dextrose will be used (50% dextrose provides 1.7 Kcal/ml).

Note: *70% dextrose solution is now available providing 2.38 Kcal/ml.*

Kcal from dextrose = total Kcal – Kcal from lipids

dextrose Kcal = 993 – 600

dextrose Kcal = 393 Kcal

$$\text{ml of dextrose needed} = \frac{\text{Kcal from dextrose}}{1.7 \text{ Kcal / ml}}$$

$$\text{ml of dextrose needed} = \frac{393 \text{ Kcal}}{1.7 \text{ Kcal / ml of } 50\% \text{ dextrose}}$$

ml of dextrose needed = 231 ml

$$\frac{231 \text{ ml}}{1} \times \frac{1.7 \text{ Kcal}}{1 \text{ ml}} = 392.7 \text{ or} \approx \textbf{393 Kcal}$$

Step 5:
To calculate the protein requirement in our example, both surgery and trauma must be considered. The protein requirement for surgery is 1 g of nitrogen for each 125 nonprotein Kcal (See table on page 162.) The requirement for trauma is 1 g of nitrogen for every 100 to 125 nonprotein Kcal. Since neither renal disease or hepatic insufficiency exist, the value for the disease state with the lowest nitrogen to Kcal ratio should be used. Trauma's ratio is lower at 1 g N for each 100 to 125 Kcal. Since the damage is extensive, a ratio of 1 g N:100 Kcal should be used.

$$\text{grams of nitrogen required} = \frac{\text{total Kcal (AER)}}{\text{Kcal to N ratio}}$$

$$\text{grams N} = \frac{993 \text{ Kcal}}{100 \text{ Kcal} / 1 \text{ g N}}$$

gram N = 9.93 g N ≈ **10 g N**

Step 6:
Commercial solutions usually express the protein content as a percentage of amino acids. Amino acid solutions are approximately 16% nitrogen. To convert the protein requirement from grams of nitrogen to grams of amino acid, divide the number of grams of amino acid required by 16% or multiply by 6.25:

$$\frac{1}{0.16} = 6.25$$

g AA required = g N required × 6.25 g AA/g N

g AA required = 10 g N × 6.25 g AA/g N

g AA required = **62.5 g AA**

Amino acid solutions are available in several strengths: 8.5% FreAmine III® and 10% Aminosyn® are common. 8.5% FreAmine III® contains 8.5 g of amino acids per 100 ml, while Aminosyn® 10% contains 10 g of amino acids per 100 ml. Determine the amount of FreAmine III® 8.5% solution required to provide 10 g of nitrogen. (Divide the number of grams of amino acids required by the concentration of the amino acid solution.)

Note: 15% Aminosyn® is now available at 15g AA/100 ml.

$$\text{quantity of AA solution required} = \frac{\text{g of AA required}}{\text{conc of AA solution}}$$

$$\text{ml of AA required} = \frac{\text{g AA required}}{8.5 \text{ g AA} / 100 \text{ ml}} \times \frac{100}{1}$$

$$\text{ml of AA required} = \frac{62.5 \text{ g AA}}{8.5 \text{ g AA} / 100 \text{ ml}} \times \frac{100}{1}$$

ml of AA required = 735 ml ≈
750 ml of 8.5% FreAmine III®

Step 7:
Fluid requirements in patients receiving TPN have been estimated at approximately 1 ml per Kcal. Fluid requirements are increased with higher ambient temperature, exercise, gestation, lactation, burns, vomiting, diarrhea, and dehydration. Fluid requirements are decreased in severe renal disease and closed head trauma.

In our example the patient has a closed head trauma. Fluids are restricted to minimize increases in intracranial pressure. The calculated AER for this patient is 993 Kcal per day; therefore, fluid requirements should be approximately 1000 ml per day. If we subtract the volume of fluids required for the administration of lipids, dextrose, and proteins from the suggested volume of 1000 ml per day, we end up with a negative number:

vol. for additives =
fluid required – (vol. of lipids + vol. of dextrose + vol. of AA)

volume = 1000 ml – (300 ml 20% lipids + 230 ml 50% dex + 750 ml 8.5% AA)

volume = – 230 ml

The fluid requirement has been exceeded by 230 ml/day. This does not mean that TPN can not be initiated but rather that additives such as electrolytes, vitamins, trace elements, and insulin (if necessary) should be kept to a minimum. Hydration should be monitored to ensure that the animal is not overhydrated.

Step 8:
As the animal's condition improves, volume allowances can be expanded to approximate normal maintenance fluids. To determine the maintenance volume for this animal, multiply the animal's weight in kilograms by the estimated fluid required in ml/kg/day. In this case you estimate fluid required at 88 ml/kg/day (40 ml/lb/day):

fluid = 20 kg × 88 ml/kg/day

fluid = 1,760 ml/day

All fluids must be considered in this requirement, including the fluid required to administer drugs (intravenous, subcutaneous, intramuscular, and oral) as well as any other intravenous fluids (e.g., D₅W, Ringer's, normal saline) and oral intake.

Step 9:

Vitamins: This dog has been hit by a car and has multiple broken bones, but it was considered healthy prior to the accident.

Lab Values: All were within normal range: Na: 140, K: 4.2, Cl: 110, BUN: 12, Cr: 0.5, glucose: 78, total protein: 6, Ca: 8.7.

Since renal function is normal, B vitamins can be added empirically to the TPN at a rate of 1 ml/L/day.

Electrolytes: Since serum electrolytes are all within normal ranges and renal function is normal, supplementation is as follows: NaCl: 130 mEq/L, KCl: 30 mEq/L. Potassium is supplemented at the higher level due to the hypertonic nature of the TPN.

Trace Elements: Since therapy is anticipated to last for only 5 to 7 days and there is no excessive GI losses requiring zinc supplementation, no trace elements are given.

Insulin: Serum glucose is within normal values so no insulin supplementation is required.

Parenteral Nutrition Worksheet for Example 2

1. Basal Energy Requirements = __662__

✓Mammals: $70 \times$ (wt in kg)$^{0.75}$

Marsupials: $49 \times$ (wt in kg)$^{0.75}$

Passerine birds: $129 \times$ (wt in kg)$^{0.75}$

Nonpasserine birds: $78 \times$ (wt in kg)$^{0.75}$

Reptiles: $10 \times$ (wt in kg)$^{0.75}$

2. Adjusted Energy Requirements = __993__
Cage rest/Nonstress starvation: 1 to 1.25 × BER
✓Postsurgery/Hepatic insufficiency: 1.25 × BER
Severe renal disease: 1.25 × BER
✓Trauma/Cancer: 1.5 × BER
Burns/Sepsis: 1.75 to 2 × BER

3. Protein Requirements = __10__ grams nitrogen

Cage rest	1 g N: 125 to150 Kcal
Nonstress starvation	1 g N: 125 to150 Kcal
✓Postsurgery	1 g N: 125 Kcal
Hepatic insufficiency	1 g N: 200 Kcal
Severe renal disease	1 g N: 200 to 500 Kcal
✓Trauma/Cancer	1 g N: 100 Kcal
Burns/Sepsis	1 g N: 80 to100 Kcal

4. Volume Requirements
a) Protein: 8.5% AA __750__ ml   (6.25 gAA/1 g N)
   max. utilization: 3 gAA/kg/day   (810 mOsm/L)
b) Lipids: 20% __300__ ml   (2 Kcal/ml)
   max. utilization: 2.5 g/kg/day   (260 mOsm/L)
c) Dextrose: 50% __230__ ml   (1.7 Kcal/ml)
   optimal rate: 7–10 g/kg/day   (2526 mOsml/L)

5. Electrolytes:
a) NaCl (4 mEq/ml) __44__ ml   (8,000 mOsm/L)
b) KCl (2 mEq/ml) __20__ ml   (4,000 mOsm/L)

6. Vitamins and Other:
MVI/B vitamins/vitamin C __1.3__ ml
Other additives: __0__ ml

7. Total Volume = __1,345__ ml   Rate: __66__ ml/hr

Osmolarity:

mOsm/L =

$$\frac{[(\text{ml } 8.5\% \text{ AA} \times 810 \text{ mOsm/L}) + (\text{ml } 20\% \text{ lipids} \times 260 \text{ mOsm/L} + ...)]}{\text{total volume}}$$

mOsm/L=

$$\frac{(750 \times 810) + (300 \times 260) + (230 + 2,526) + (44 \times 8000) + (20 + 4000)}{1,345}$$

$$\text{mOsm/L} = \frac{1,698,480}{1,345}$$

mOsm/L = **1,263**

Order: Total parenteral nutrition (TPN) containing 750 ml 8.5% AA, 300 ml 20% lipids, 230 ml 50% dextrose, 44 ml of 4 mEq/ml NaCl, 20 ml of 2 mEq/ml KCl, and 1.3 ml B vitamins should be infused via a central line at 68 ml/hr.

★ **Example 3:** *A 44 lb dog has been vomiting and unable to eat for 10 days. Develop a TPN treatment for this dog.*

Step 1:
Choose the BER equation for mammals.

BER for mammals = $70 \times (\text{wt in kg})^{0.75}$

Convert the weight from pounds to kilograms:

$$\frac{44 \text{ lb}}{1} \times \frac{1 \text{ kg}}{2.2 \text{ lb}} = 20 \text{ kg}$$

Insert the weight and calculate the BER.

BER = $70 \times (20)^{0.75}$

BER = 70 × 9.46 Kcal/day

BER = **662.2 Kcal/day**

Step 2:
Clinical pathology findings include Na: 132, K: 3.4, Cl: 110, BUN: 22, creatinine: 1.9, glucose: 78, bicarbonate: 26.

Sodium, potassium, magnesium, and chloride are lost when vomiting is present. Vomiting often results in alkalosis as evidenced by an increased bicarbonate level. The BUN and creatinine are elevated, but the increases are suggestive of prerenal azotemia.

Gross electrolyte abnormalities should be corrected before initiating TPN, but potassium should be administered cautiously when renal disease is present.

A 500 ml bolus of normal saline is administered followed by 500 ml of saline and 20 mg of Lasix®. Urine output increases. Normal saline with 20 mEq KCl per liter will be administered at maintenance levels.

Step 3:
If normal maintenance fluid requirements for dogs are estimated at 40 ml per pound per day, determine the maintenance volume for this animal by multiplying the animal's weight in pounds by 40 ml per pound per day:

44 lb × 40 ml/lb/day = 1,760 ml/day

This is a maintenance volume for 24 hours; to determine the rate of administration, divide the volume in milliliters per day by 24 hours per day. The result is the administration rate in milliliters per hour:

$$\text{ml / hr} = \frac{\text{volume (ml / day)}}{24 \text{ hours / day}}$$

$$ml / hr = \frac{1,760 \ ml / day}{24 \ hour / day}$$

ml/hr = **73.3 ml/hr**

Step 4:
The BER was previously calculated at 662 Kcal/day. The adjusted energy requirement (AER) can now be calculated, taking into account that this animal has been anorexic.

The AER for starvation is 1.25 × BER, when no other disease states are present. Using the AER for starvation, we calculate the adjusted energy expenditure to be

AER = 1.25 × BER

AER = 1.25 × 662 Kcal/day

AER = 827.5 Kcal/day ≈ **830 Kcal/day**

Step 5:
If 40% of the calories are to be provided by lipids, multiply AER by percentage of calories to obtain the number of Kcal provided from lipids.

830 Kcal × 0.4 = 332 Kcal

$$ml \ of \ lipids = \frac{Kcal \ from \ lipids}{2 \ Kcal \ / \ ml \ of \ 20\% \ lipids}$$

$$ml \ of \ lipids = \frac{332 \ Kcal}{2 \ Kcal \ / \ ml \ of \ 20\% \ lipids}$$

ml of lipids =166 ml ≈ 170 ml of 20% lipids ≈ **340 Kcal**

Step 6:

If 40% of nonprotein Kcal are coming from lipids, then 60% (100 – 40%) should be obtained in the form of dextrose. Unless otherwise specified, 50% dextrose will be used. (50% dextrose provides 1.7 Kcal/ml.)

Kcal from dextrose = total Kcal – Kcal from lipids

Kcal from dextrose = 830 – 340

Kcal from dextrose = 490 Kcal

$$\text{ml from dextrose} = \frac{\text{Kcal from dextrose}}{1.7 \text{ Kcal / ml}}$$

$$\text{ml from dextrose} = \frac{490 \text{ Kcal}}{1.7 \text{ Kcal / ml of } 50\% \text{ dex}}$$

ml from dextrose = 288 ml ≈ 300 ml of 50% dex ≈ **510 Kcal**

Step 7:

The protein requirement for nonstress starvation is 1 g of nitrogen for every 125 to 150 nonprotein calories. To calculate the protein required, divide the AER by 1 g N:150 Kcal:

$$\text{grams of nitrogen required} = \frac{\text{total calories (AER)}}{\text{Kcal to N ratio}}$$

$$\text{nitrogen required} = \frac{830 \text{ Kcal}}{150 \text{ Kcal / 1 g N}}$$

nitrogen required = 5.53 g N

Commercial solutions usually express the protein content as a percentage of amino acids. Amino acid solutions are approximately 16% nitrogen. To convert the protein requirement from grams of nitrogen to grams of amino acids, divide the number of grams of amino acids required by 16% or multiply by 6.25:

$$\text{g AA required} = \frac{1}{0.16} = 6.25$$

g AA required = g N required × 6.25 g AA/g N

g AA required = 5.5 g N × 6.25 g AA/g N

g AA required = 34.375 g AA

Amino acid solutions are available in several strengths. 8.5% FreAmine III® and 10% Aminosyn® are common. 8.5% FreAmine III® contains 8.5 g of amino acids per 100 ml, while Aminosyn® 10% contains 10 g of amino acids per 100 ml. Determine the amount of Aminosyn® 10% solution required to provide 21 g of amino acids. (Divide the number of grams of amino acids required by the concentration of the amino acid solution.)

$$\text{quantity of AA solution} = \frac{\text{grams of AA required}}{\text{conc of AA solution}}$$

$$\text{ml of AA} = \left(\frac{\text{g AA required}}{10\text{g AA}/100 \text{ ml}}\right)$$

$$\text{ml of AA} = \frac{34 \text{ g AA}}{10 \text{ g AA}/100 \text{ ml}}$$

ml of AA = **340 ml of 10% Aminosyn®**

Step 8:
Fluid requirements in patients receiving TPN have been estimated at approximately 1 ml per Kcal. Fluid requirements are increased with higher ambient temperature,

exercise, gestation, lactation, burns, vomiting, diarrhea, and dehydration. Fluid requirements are decreased in severe renal disease and closed head trauma.

fluid requirements = 1 ml per Kcal of nutrients supplied
AER = 830 Kcal, therefore fluid required ≈ 830 ml

The volume of fluids available for additives is determined by subtracting the volume of fluids required for the administration of lipids, dextrose, and proteins from the suggested volume of 830 ml per day.

volume available =

fluid requirements – (lipid volume + dextrose volume + AA volume)

volume =

830 ml – (170 ml 20% lipids + 300 ml 50% dex + 340 ml 10% AA)

volume = 20 ml

The fluid requirement is 20 ml/day. Hydration should be monitored to ensure that the animal is not overhydrated but volume allowances can be expanded to approximate normal maintenance fluid levels. Normal maintenance fluid levels for dogs are estimated at 40 ml per pound per day. To determine the maintenance volume for this animal, multiply the animal's weight in pounds by 40 ml per pound per day:

44 lb × 40 ml/lb/day = **1,760 ml/day**

The maintenance volume must include all fluids that will be administered including fluids containing drugs, other intravenous fluids (e.g., D$_5$W, lactated Ringer's, normal saline) and any oral intake. Since the TPN will provide 810 ml/day, 950 ml needs to be provided by additional fluids (e.g., 0.9% NaCl) or oral intake. A peripheral line is inserted and 1 L of normal saline is administered per day.

Step 9:

Vitamins: This dog currently has laboratory values within the normal range so that B vitamins can be added empirically to the TPN at a rate of 1 ml/L/day. If renal function is compromised, the administration of water soluble vitamins should be restricted.

Electrolytes: Because serum electrolytes are now within normal ranges and renal function is normal, supplementation should be as follows: NaCl 130 meq/L, KCl 30 meq/L. Potassium should be supplemented at the higher level due to the hypertonic nature of the TPN. When hypertonic solutions are administered, potassium is often driven intracellularly resulting in lower plasma levels. To correct for this effect, additional potassium is administered and adjustments are made based on subsequent laboratory values.

Trace Elements: Most TPN therapies last for only 5 to 7 days. Supplementation of trace elements may not be required unless therapy exceeds 2 to 3 weeks or there is excessive GI loss (e.g., diarrhea). If diarrhea or other causes of GI loss are present, zinc supplementation sould be initiated. In this case, no trace elements should be given.

Insulin: Serum glucose is within normal values, so no insulin is required.

Parenteral Nutrition Worksheet for Example 3

1. Basal Energy Requirements = __662__

✓Mammals: $70 \times (\text{wt in kg})^{0.75}$

Marsupials: $49 \times (\text{wt in kg})^{0.75}$

Passerine birds: $129 \times (\text{wt in kg})^{0.75}$

Nonpasserine birds: $78 \times (\text{wt in kg})^{0.75}$

Reptiles: $10 \times (\text{wt in kg})^{0.75}$

2. Adjusted Energy Requirements = __830__
✓Cage rest/Nonstress starvation: 1 to 1.25 × BER
Postsurgery/Hepatic insufficiency: 1.25 × BER
Severe renal disease: 1.25 × BER
Trauma/Cancer: 1.5 × BER
Burns/Sepsis: 1.75 to 2 × BER

3. Protein Requirements = __5.5__ grams nitrogen
✓Cage rest	1 g N: 125 to150 Kcal
Nonstress starvation	1 g N: 125 to150 Kcal
Postsurgery	1 g N: 125 Kcal
Hepatic insufficiency	1 g N: 200 Kcal
Severe renal disease	1 g N: 200 to 500 Kcal
Trauma/Cancer	1 g N: 100 Kcal
Burns/Sepsis	1 g N: 80 to 100 Kcal

4. Volume Requirements
a) Protein: 10% AA __340__ ml   (6.25 gAA/1 g N)
   max. utilization: 3 gAA/kg/day   (810 mOsm/L)
b) Lipids: 20% __170__ ml   (2 Kcal/ml)
   max. utilization: 2.5 g/kg/day   (260 mOsm/L)
c) Dextrose: 50% __300__ ml   (1.7 Kcal/ml)
   optimal rate: 7–10 g/kg/day   (2526 mOsml/L)

5. Electrolytes:
a) NaCl (4 mEq/ml) __29__ ml   (8,000 mOsm/L)
b) KCl (2 mEq/ml) __15__ ml   (4,000 mOsm/L)

6. Vitamins and Other:
MVI/B vitamins/vitamin C __1__ ml
Other additives: __0__ ml

7. Total Volume = __885__ ml   Rate: __44__ ml/hr
If TPN contains lipids give over 20 hours; if not, give
over 24 hours.

Osmolarity =

$$\frac{[(ml \; AA \times 810 \; mOsm / L) + (ml \; 20\% \; lipids \times 260 \; mOsm / L) + \ldots]}{total \; volume}$$

mOsm/L =

$$\frac{(340 \times 810) + (170 \times 200) + (300 \times 2,526) + (29 \times 8,000) + (15 \times 4,000)}{885 \; ml}$$

$$mOsm/L = \frac{59,200}{885}$$

mOsm/L = **1,536**

Order: TPN containing 340 ml 10% AA, 170 ml 20% lipids, 300 ml 50% dextrose, 29 ml of 4 mEq/ml NaCl, 15 ml of 2 mEq/ml KCl, and 1 ml B vitamins to be infused via a central line at 44 ml/hr.

★ **Example 4:** *A 2 kg Canada goose is presented to the clinic with possible lead toxicity. Radiographs reveal several metallic densities in the intestine. You place the animal on Ca-EDTA and decide to remove what appears to be a damaged section of tissue. The surgery goes well but the goose will be given nothing per os (NPO) for several days to provide the intestine time to heal. Calculate the BER, AER, and volumes of 50% dextrose and 10% Aminosyn® required to meet this animal's nutritional needs.*

Step 1:
Calculate the BER for the Canada goose using the equation for nonpasserine birds. (If you do not have a calculator available with a y^x function key, see Appendix J.)

BER for nonpasserines = $78 \times$ (wt in kg)$^{0.75}$

BER= 78×1.68 = **131 Kcal/day**

Step 2:
Adjusted energy requirements are based on disease states present and stage of life. The AER for post-surgery is 1.25 × BER (See p. 151).

AER = 1.25 × BER

AER= 1.25 × 131 Kcal/day

AER= 163.75 ≈ 164 Kcal/day

A mixed energy source is usually preferred; however, dextrose has been successfully used as a sole energy source. Calculate the amount of 50% dextrose needed to provide the AER (50% dextrose = 1.7 Kcal/ml):

$$\text{vol of 50\% dex required} = \frac{\text{AER}}{\text{caloric value of 50\% dex}}$$

$$\text{volume dextrose} = \frac{164}{1.7 \text{ Kcal / ml}}$$

volume dextrose = 96.47 ml ≈ **100 ml**

Step 3:
Protein requirements following surgery are 1 g N for every 125 Kcal (See p.162). To determine the number of grams of nitrogen required, divide the AER by 125 Kcal:

$$\text{grams of N required} = \frac{\text{AER}}{125 \text{ Kcal}}$$

$$\text{g N} = \frac{164 \text{ Kcal}}{125 \text{ Kcal}}$$

g N = 1.3 g N

To convert from grams of nitrogen to grams of amino acids multiply by 6.25:

g AA = 1.3 g N × 6.25

g AA = 8.125 g amino acids

To determine the volume of 10% Aminosyn® required to provide 8.125 g, divide by 10 g/100 ml (10% Aminosyn® contains 10 g of amino acids per 100 ml):

$$\text{volume} = \frac{8.125 \text{ g}}{10 \text{ g}/100 \text{ ml}}$$

$$\text{volume} = \frac{8.125}{10} \times \frac{100}{1}$$

volume = 81.25 ≈ **80 ml 10% Aminosyn®**

This animal's protein and calorie requirements can be met using 100 ml of 50% dextrose and 80 ml of 10% Aminosyn®. The resulting solution is very hypertonic and should be administered in the femoral vein or intraosseously.

Parenteral Nutrition Worksheet for Example 4

1. Basal Energy Requirements = __131__

Mammals: $70 \times (\text{wt in kg})^{0.75}$

Marsupials: $49 \times (\text{wt in kg})^{0.75}$

Passerine birds: $129 \times (\text{wt in kg})^{0.75}$

✓Nonpasserine birds: $78 \times (\text{wt in kg})^{0.75}$

Reptiles: $10 \times (\text{wt in kg})0.75$

2. Adjusted Energy Requirements = __164__

Cage rest/Nonstress starvation: 1 to 1.25 × BER

✓Postsurgery/Hepatic insufficiency: 1.25 × BER

Severe renal disease: 1.25 × BER

Trauma/Cancer: 1.5 × BER

Burns/Sepsis: 1.75 to 2 × BER

3. Protein Requirements = __1.3__ grams nitrogen

Cage rest	1 g N: 125–150 Kcal
Nonstress starvation	1 g N: 125–150 Kcal
✓Postsurgery	1 g N: 125 Kcal
Hepatic insufficiency	1 g N: 200 Kcal
Severe renal disease	1 g N: 200–500 Kcal
Trauma/Cancer	1 g N: 100 Kcal
Burns/Sepsis	1 g N: 80–100 Kcal

4. Volume Requirements
a) Protein: 10% AA __80__ ml   (6.25 gAA/1 g N)
    max. utilization: 3 gAA/kg/day   (810 mOsm/L)
b) Lipids: 20% _____ ml   (2 Kcal/ml)
    max. utilization: 2.5 g/kg/day   (260 mOsm/L)
c) Dextrose: 50% __100__ ml   (1.7 Kcal/ml)
    optimal rate: 7–10 g/kg/day   (2526 mOsml/L)

5. Electrolytes:
a) NaCl (4 mEq/ml) _____ ml   (8,000 mOsm/L)
b) KCl (2 mEq/ml) _____ ml   (4,000 mOsm/L)

6. Vitamins and Other:
MVI/B vitamins/vitamin C _____ ml
Other additives: _____ ml

7. Total Volume = __180__ ml   Rate: __8__ ml/hr
If TPN contains lipids give over 20 hours, if not, give
over 24 hours.

Osmolarity =

$$\frac{[(ml\ AA \times 810\ mOsm / L) + (ml\ 20\%\ lipids \times 260\ mOsm / L) + ...]}{total\ volume}$$

$$mOsm/L = \frac{(80 \times 810) + (100 \times 2{,}526)}{180}$$

$$mOsm/L = \frac{317,400}{180}$$

mOsm/L = **1,763**

Order: TPN containing 80 ml 10% AA and 100 ml 50% dextrose to be infused via a central line at 8 ml/hr.

★ **Example 5:** *A 70 lb foal is presented to the clinic with a 5 day history of not eating. It has been receiving 1 L of 5% dextrose each day. What is the nutritional content of this fluid? Calculate the number of grams of dextrose in this preparation:*

By definition,
5% dextrose = 5 g/100 ml
1 L = 1000 ml

Step 1:
grams of dextrose = conc of commercial prep. (g/100 ml) × volume administered (ml)

$$g\ dextrose = \frac{1000\ \cancel{ml}}{1} \times \frac{5\ g}{100\ \cancel{ml}}$$

g dextrose = 50 g

Each gram of carbohydrate contains 3.4 Kcal. Thus, 50 g × 3.4 Kcal/g = **170 Kcal**

Step 2:
What percent of a 70 lb foal's BER is 170 Kcal?

Convert the weight from pounds to kilograms (See Appendix G):

$$\frac{70 \cancel{lb}}{1} \times \frac{1 \text{ kg}}{2.2 \cancel{lb}} = 31.8 \text{ kg}$$

Insert the weight in kilograms into the BER equation for mammals:

BER for mammals = $70 \times (31.8)^{0.75}$

BER for mammals = 70×13.39

BER for mammals = **937.3 Kcal**

Step 3:
Divide the caloric content of the fluid by the BER:

$$\frac{170 \text{ Kcal}}{937.3 \text{ Kcal}} \times 100\% = 18.1\%$$

The animal is lethargic and losing weight. You decide to place this animal on TPN. Using the adjusted energy requirement for starvation, calculate this animal's adjusted energy requirement.

AER (starvation) = $1.25 \times$ BER

AER = 1.25×937.3

AER = **1171.6 Kcal/day**

Step 4:
Using a mixed energy source is usually preferred, but you have no lipids in the pharmacy. Calculate the amount of 50% dextrose needed to provide the AER. (Remember that 50% dextrose provides 1.7 Kcal/ml.)

$$50\% \text{ dextrose needed in ml} = \frac{\text{AER in Kcal}}{1.7 \text{ Kcal / ml}}$$

$$\text{dextrose volume} = \frac{1171.6 \text{ Kcal}}{1.7 \text{ Kcal / ml}}$$

dextrose volume = 689 ml ≈ **700 ml**

Step 5:
The protein requirement for starvation is 1 g of nitrogen for every 125 to 150 Kcal (See table pg. 162). Using the value 1 g N:125 Kcal, calculate the volume of 8.5% Aminosyn® required to provide the nitrogen requirements for this patient.

$$\text{g N} = \frac{\text{AER}}{\text{Kcal / g N ratio}}$$

$$\text{g N} = \frac{1171.6 \text{ Kcal}}{100 \text{ Kcal / 1 g N}}$$

g N = 11.72 g N ≈ 12 g N

g AA = g N × (6.25 g AA/g N)

g AA = 12 × 6.25

g AA = 75 g AA

$$\text{volume Aminosyn® required} = \frac{\text{g AA}}{\text{conc of AA in g / 100 ml}}$$

$$\text{volume} = \frac{75 \text{ g AA}}{8.5 \text{ g AA / 100 ml}}$$

volume = **882 ml**

Thus, the protein and calorie requirements of this animal can be met using 700 ml of a 50% dextrose solution and 880 ml of 8.5% FreAmine III®. This is a very hypertonic solution and should only be administered through a central line. Electrolytes and vitamins should be supplemented based on laboratory values for this patient and the catheter site monitored for signs of infection or irritation.

Parenteral Nutrition Worksheet for Example 5

1. Basal Energy Requirements = 937.3
✓Mammals: 70 × (wt in kg)$^{0.75}$
Marsupials: 49 × (wt in kg)$^{0.75}$
Passerine birds: 129 × (wt in kg)$^{0.75}$
Nonpasserine birds: 78 × (wt in kg)$^{0.75}$
Reptiles: 10 × (wt in kg)$^{0.75}$

2. Adjusted Energy Requirements = 1,171.6
✓Cage rest/Nonstress starvation: 1 to 1.25 × BER
Postsurgery/Hepatic insufficiency: 1.25 × BER
Severe renal disease: 1.25 × BER
Trauma/Cancer: 1.5 × BER
Burns/Sepsis: 1.75 to 2 × BER

3. Protein Requirements = 11.72 grams nitrogen

Cage rest	1 g N: 125 to150 Kcal
✓Nonstress starvation	1 g N: 125 to 150 Kcal
Postsurgery	1 g N: 125 Kcal
Hepatic insufficiency	1 g N: 200 Kcal
Severe renal disease	1 g N: 200 to 500 Kcal
Trauma/Cancer	1 g N: 100 Kcal
Burns/Sepsis	1 g N: 80 to 100 Kcal

4. Volume Requirements
a) Protein: 8.5% AA 880 (882) ml (6.25 g AA/1 g N)
   max. utilization: 3 g AA/kg/day   (810 mOsm/L)
b) Lipids: 20% _____ ml   (2 Kcal/ml)
   max. utilization: 2.5 g/kg/day   (260 mOsm/L)
c) Dextrose: 50% 700 (689) ml   (1.7 Kcal/ml)
   optimal rate: 7–10 g/kg/day   (2526 mOsml/L)

5. Electrolytes:
a) NaCl (4 mEq/ml) _____ ml   (8,000 mOsm/L)
b) KCl (2 mEq/ml) _____ ml   (4,000 mOsm/L)

6. Vitamins and Other:
MVI/B vitamins/vitamin C _____ ml
Other additives: __0__ ml

7. Total Volume = __1,580__ ml   Rate: __66__ ml/hr
If TPN contains lipids give over 20 hours; if not, give over 24 hours.

Osmolarity =

$$\frac{[(ml\ AA \times 810\ mOsm\ /\ L) + (ml\ 20\%\ lipids \times 260\ mOsm\ /\ L) + ...]}{total\ volume}$$

$$mOsm\ /\ L = \frac{(880 \times 810) + (700 \times 2,562)}{1,580}$$

$$mOsm/L = \frac{2,506,200}{1,580}$$

mOsm/L = **1,586**

Order: TPN containing 880 ml 8.5% AA and 700 ml 50% dextrose, to be infused via a central line at 66 ml/hr.

★ **Example 6:** *A 1000 lb, 23-year-old horse is presented to the clinic with choke. Surgery was required to remove the obstruction. Tissue around the esophagus was necrotic and the animal is not to receive food for 7 to 10 days post-surgery. TPN is initiated using 500 ml $D_{50}W$, 1000 ml 8.5% amino acids, and 500 ml 20% lipids + electrolytes. What percent of the BER does this regimen meet?*

Step 1:
Choose the BER equation for mammals:
BER for mammals = $70 \times (kg)^{0.75}$

Convert the body weight from pounds to kilograms:

$$\frac{1000 \ \cancel{lb}}{1} \times \frac{1 \ kg}{2.2 \ \cancel{lb}} = 454 \ kg$$

Calculate the BER:

BER = $70 \times (454)^{0.75}$

BER = 70×98.35

BER = **6,884.8 Kcal**

Step 2:
Calculate the amount of nonprotein calories contained in this regimen:

50% dextrose = 1.7 Kcal/ml from dextrose

1.7 Kcal/ml × 500 ml = 850 Kcal

20% lipids = 2 Kcal/ml

2 Kcal/ml × 500 ml = 1000 Kcal from lipids

total nonprotein calories = 850 dextrose + 1000 lipids

total nonprotein calories = **1,850 Kcal**

Step 3:
Calculate the percentage of the BER that this regimen meets:

$$\text{percentage of BER} = \frac{\text{Kcal administered}}{\text{calc. BER}}$$

$$\% \text{ BER} = \frac{1850 \text{ Kcal}}{6884.8 \text{ Kcal}} \times 100\%$$

% BER = **26.9%**

Step 4:
How much protein is provided by the 1000 ml of 8.5% amino acid solution?

By definition, 8.5% = 8.5 g/100 ml

$$\frac{1000 \text{ ml}}{1} \times \frac{8.5 \text{ g}}{100 \text{ ml}} = 85 \text{ g amino acids}$$

6.25 g amino acids = 1 g nitrogen

$$\frac{85 \text{ g}}{1} \times \frac{1 \text{ g N}}{6.25 \text{ g AA}} = 13.6 \text{ g nitrogen}$$

Parenteral Nutrition Worksheet for Example 6
1. Basal Energy Requirements = <u>6,884.8</u>
✓Mammals: $70 \times (\text{wt in kg})^{0.75}$
Marsupials: $49 \times (\text{wt in kg})^{0.75}$
Passerine birds: $129 \times (\text{wt in kg})^{0.75}$
Nonpasserine birds: $78 \times (\text{wt in kg})^{0.75}$
Reptiles: $10 \times (\text{wt in kg})^{0.75}$

2. Adjusted Energy Requirements = <u>8,606</u>
Cage rest/Nonstress starvation: 1 to 1.25 × BER
✓Postsurgery/Hepatic insufficiency: 1.25 × BER
Severe renal disease: 1.25 × BER
Trauma/Cancer: 1.5 × BER
Burns/Sepsis: 1.75 to 2 × BER
Growth: 1.5 to 2 × BER

3. Protein Requirements = __13.6__ grams nitrogen

Cage rest	1 g N: 125 to 150 Kcal
Nonstress starvation	1 g N: 125 to 150 Kcal
✓Postsurgery	1 g N: 125 Kcal
Hepatic insufficiency	1 g N: 200 Kcal
Severe renal disease	1 g N: 200 to 500 Kcal
Trauma/Cancer	1 g N: 100 Kcal
Burns/Sepsis	1 g N: 80 to 100 Kcal
Growth:	1.5 to 2 × BER

4. Volume Requirements

a) Protein: 8.5% AA __1000__ ml (6.25 gAA/1 g N)
   max. utilization: 3 gAA/kg/day (810 mOsm/L)
b) Lipids: 20% __500__ ml (2 Kcal/ml)
   max. utilization: 2.5 g/kg/day (260 mOsm/L)
c) Dextrose: 50% __500__ ml (1.7 Kcal/ml)
   optimal rate: 7–10 g/kg/day (2,526 mOsml/L)

5. Electrolytes:

a) NaCl (4 mEq/ml) _____ ml (8,000 mOsm/L)
b) KCl (2 mEq/ml) _____ ml (4,000 mOsm/L)

6. Vitamins and Other:

MVI/B vitamins/vitamin C _____ ml
Other additives: _____ ml

7. Total Volume = __2,000__ ml   Rate: _____ ml/hr
If TPN contains lipids give over 20 hours, if not, give
over 24 hours.

Osmolarity=

$$\frac{[(\text{ml AA} \times 810\,\text{mOsm} / L) + (\text{ml 20\% lipids} \times 260\,\text{mOsm} / L) + ...]}{\text{total volume}}$$

$$\text{mOsm} = \frac{(1000 \times 810) + (500 \times 260) + (500 \times 2{,}526)}{2{,}000}$$

$$\text{mOsm} = \frac{2{,}203{,}000}{2{,}000}$$

mOsm/L = **1,101**

Toxicology

Formula Summary

ppm = $g/1,000,000$ ml = mg/L = mcg/ml

mg %= mg/100 ml

mg/dl = mg/100 ml

mg/ml = mg % × 100

LD_{50} = lethal dose (amount) that will kill approximately 50% of a group of animals

$$\text{blood level} = \frac{\text{amt ingested} \times (\% \text{ sol} /100) \times \text{specific gravity}}{\text{Vd} \times \text{wt}}$$

where Vd= volume of distribution of the substance

conc (%) × vol (ml) = conc (g/100 ml) × vol (ml)

drug required for maintenance dosing = (animal's wt in lb × 1 kg/2.2 lb) × maintenance dose (mg/kg) × duration of therapy in days × 24 hours/day × dosing frequency (e.g., 1 dose/unknown hours)

$$\text{volume required (ml)} = \frac{\text{total dose (ml)}}{\text{concentration (mg / ml)}}$$

Toxicology Examples

★ **Example:** *Lead plasma levels in a dog are found to be 400 mcg/dl. (Normal levels are 50–150 mcg/dl). You find a reference that recommends chelation with Desferal® for lead levels greater than 5 mg %. Convert the measured lead level from mcg/dl to mg % (mg % = mg/100 ml) to determine if this dog requires Desferal®.*

Step 1:
Begin by converting from micrograms to milligrams
(See Appendix G):

$$\frac{400 \; \cancel{mcg}}{1 \; dl} \times \frac{1 \; mg}{1000 \; \cancel{mcg}} = 0.4 \; mg \, / \, dl$$

Step 2:
Convert from deciliters to milliliters:

$$\frac{0.4 \; mg}{1 \; \cancel{dl}} \times \frac{1 \; \cancel{dl}}{100 \; ml} = 0.4 \; mg \, / \, 100 \; ml$$

By definition (mg/100 ml) is the same as (mg %).

Therefore, 0.4 mg/100 ml = 0.4 mg %

Since the lead plasma level in the dog was less than 5 mg %, you determine that chelation with Desferal® is not necessary.

★ **Example:** *A 4-month-old, 2.2 kg female Pomeranian is presented with acute anorexia, vomiting, salivation, icteric mucous membranes, and anemia. Four round, flat objects the size of pennies are noted on radiographs. Serum zinc concentration is found to be 28.8 mg/L using atomic absorption spectrophotometry. Ingestion of two pennies has been reported as fatal in a 5 kg dog; thus, surgery will be performed. Convert the serum zinc concentration from mg/L to ppm.*

Step 1:
Since ppm can also be defined as g/1,000,000 ml, convert to common units (g and ml). To convert the numerator from milligrams to grams, multiply by the factor 1 g = 1000 mg (See Appendix G):

$$\frac{28.8 \text{ mg}}{1 \text{ L}} \times \frac{1 \text{ g}}{1000 \text{ mg}} = 0.0288 \text{ g / L}$$

Step 2:
Convert the denominator from liters to milliliters by using the fact that 1 L = 1000 ml (See Appendix G):

$$\frac{0.0288 \text{ g}}{1 \text{ L}} \times \frac{1 \text{ L}}{1000 \text{ ml}} = \frac{0.0288 \text{ g}}{1000 \text{ ml}}$$

Step 3:
By definition, ppm = g/1,000,000 ml. So set up a ratio:

$$\frac{0.0288 \text{ g}}{1000 \text{ ml}} = \frac{\text{unknown g}}{1,000,000 \text{ ml}}$$

Cross multiply to solve the equation.

unknown g × 1000 = 0.0288 × 1,000,000

$$\text{unknown g} = \frac{28,800}{1000}$$

unknown g = 28.8

Therefore:

$$\frac{28.8 \text{ mg}}{1000 \text{ ml}} \times \frac{1000 \text{ g}}{1 \text{ mg}} \times \frac{1}{1000} = \frac{28.8 \text{ g}}{1,000,000 \text{ ml}} = 28.8 \text{ ppm}$$

★ **Example:** *Charcoal has been used to absorb potential toxins from the gastrointestinal tract when gastric lavage or induction of vomiting is not recommended. Determine the amount of charcoal required to treat a 67 lb potbellied pig at 2 g of charcoal per kilogram of body weight.*

Step 1:
Convert the weight of the pig from pounds to kilograms (See Appendix G):

wt (kg) = wt (lb) × 1 kg/2.2 lb

$$wt \ (kg) = 67 \, \cancel{lb} \times \frac{1 \ kg}{2.2 \, \cancel{lb}} = 30.45 \ kg$$

Step 2:
To determine the amount of charcoal required, multiply the dose required in grams per kilogram by the weight of the animal in kilograms:

g charcoal = wt (kg) × 2 g charcoal/kg of weight

g charcoal = 30.45 kg × 2 g/kg

g charcoal = 60.9 g

Step 3:
If the charcoal is to be administered in 3 ml of water per gram of charcoal, how much water is required? Determine the amount of water required by multiplying the dose required in ml of water per gram of charcoal by the number of grams of charcoal needed:

vol of H_2O = dose (ml/g) of charcoal × g of charcoal

vol of H_2O = 3 ml water/g of charcoal × 60.9 g charcoal

volume of water = **182.7 ml**

★ **Example:** *Deferoxamine is used in the treatment of iron overload or intoxication. 100 parts of* *deferoxamine by weight can bind 8.5 parts by weight of ferric iron. A dose of 20–40 mg/kg intramuscularly or intravenously is used for dogs. How much deferoxamine should be used to treat a 43 kg dog that is showing signs of iron toxicity?*

Multiply the weight of the animal in kilograms by the dose in milligrams per kilogram. Since a range is suggested, the lower and upper ends of the range should be calculated and the dosage determined by the level of clinical toxicity:

dose required = wt (kg) × dose (mg/kg)

dosage at 20 mg/kg = 43 kg × 20 mg/kg = 860 mg

dosage at 40 mg/kg = 43 kg × 40 mg/kg = 1,720 mg

dosage range = **860 to 1,720 mg**

★ **Example**: *Dimercaprol (BAL) has been used to treat arsenic poisoning in a variety of mammals. A dose of 4 mg/kg IM every 4 hours until recovery is used to treat arsenic poisoning in a dog. If the dog is a 92 lb shepherd, how much dimercaprol is needed per dose?*

Step 1:
Covert the weight of the animal from pounds to kilogram (See Appendix G):

wt (kg) = wt (lb) × 1 kg/2.2 lb

$$\text{wt (kg)} = 92 \, \cancel{\text{lb}} \times \frac{1 \text{ kg}}{2.2 \, \cancel{\text{lb}}} = 41.8 \text{ kg}$$

Step 2:

Multiply the weight of the animal (kg) by the dose (mg/kg):

dose required = wt (kg) × dose (mg/kg)

dose required = 41.8 kg × 4 mg/kg

dose required = **167 mg of BAL per dose**

★ **Example:** *Methylene blue has been used to treat nitrate toxicity in cattle at a dose of 8.8 mg/kg intravenously in a 1% solution. If you are summoned to a herd of cattle experiencing nitrate toxicity, how much of a 1% methylene blue solution would you need to give each cow if the average weight is 1,100 lb?*

Step 1:

Covert the weight from pounds to kilograms:

wt (kg) = wt (lb) × 1 kg/2.2 lb

$$\text{wt (kg)} = 1{,}100 \, \cancel{\text{lb}} \times \frac{1 \text{ kg}}{2.2 \, \cancel{\text{lb}}}$$

wt (kg)= 500 kg

Step 2:

To determine the dose in milligrams that each animal should receive, multiply the dose required (mg/kg) by the weight of the average animal (kg):

dose required = dose (mg/kg) × wt (kg)

dose required = 8.8 mg/kg × 500 kg

dose required = 4,400 mg

Step 3:
To determine the amount of 1% methylene blue solution that should be administered to each affected animal, divide the dose required in milligrams by the concentration of the solution (mg/ml).

By definition,
1% = 1 g/100 ml = 1000 mg/100 ml = 10 mg/ml

$$\text{dose (ml)} = \frac{\text{dose required (mg)}}{\text{concentration (mg / ml)}}$$

$$\text{dose} = \frac{4,400 \text{ mg}}{10 \text{ mg / ml}}$$

dose = **440 ml**

★ **Example:** *D-Penicillamine (Cuprimine®) has been used for copper-associated hepatopathy in dogs at a dose of 10–15 mg/kg orally q12h on an empty stomach. What dose is required for a 22 kg dog?*

Multiply the animal's weight in kilogram by the dose in milligrams per kilogram. Since a dosage range has been expressed, a calculation should be done to determine the high and low ends of the range:

dose required (mg) = wt (kg) × dose (mg/kg)

dosage at 10 mg/kg = 22 kg × 10 mg/kg = 220 mg

dosage at 15 mg/kg = to 22 kg × 15 mg/kg = 330 mg

dosage range = **220 to 330 mg**

Since Cuprimine® is available as a 250 mg tablet, one tablet should be given every 12 hours.

★ **Example:** *Pralidoxime (2-PAM) can be used to treat organophosphate toxicity. If a dose of 20 mg/kg is prescribed for a 6 lb cat that was dipped in an organophosphate dip 12 hours ago, how much 2-PAM will be needed per dose?*

Step 1:
Convert the weight of the cat from pounds to kilograms:

wt (kg) = wt (lb) × 1 kg/2.2 lb

$$\text{wt (kg)} = 6\,\cancel{\text{lb}} \times \frac{1\ \text{kg}}{2.2\ \cancel{\text{lb}}}$$

wt (kg) = 2.7 kg

Step 2:
Multiply the dose required (in mg/kg) by the weight of the animal in kilograms to determine the amount of 2-PAM needed per dose:

dose required (mg) = dose (mg/kg) × wt (kg)

dose = 20 mg/kg × 2.7 kg

dose = 54.5 kg

★ **Example**: *A 12.3 kg dog died after ingesting 2 lb of milk chocolate, which was estimated to contain approximately 1,600 mg of theobromine. The potentially lethal dose of caffeine or theobromine is 100–250 mg/kg or about 2 ounces of milk chocolate per kilogram of body weight.*

A lethal serum concentration of theobromine has been reported to be 133 mg/L. Convert this lethal serum concentration to a) mg/ml, b) mg %, c) mg/dl, d) ppm, and e) mcg/ml. Remember to convert to common units.

a) Convert 133 mg/L to mg/ml by using common units. In this problem only the denominator needs to be converted because the numerator is and will remain in milligrams. To convert the denominator from liters to milliliters, recall that 1 liter = 1000 milliliters:

$$\frac{133 \text{ mg}}{1 \cancel{L}} \times \frac{1 \cancel{L}}{1000 \text{ ml}} = \frac{0.133 \text{ mg}}{\text{ml}} = 0.1333 \text{ mg} / \text{ml}$$

b) To convert mg/L to mg %, recall that by definition mg % is the same as mg/100 ml. In step a) you have already determined that 133 mg/L = 0.133 mg/ml. Take this information and convert it to mg/100 ml by using a ratio:

$$\frac{0.133 \text{ mg}}{1 \text{ ml}} = \frac{\text{unknown mg}}{100 \text{ ml}} = \text{mg} \%$$

Cross multiply to solve the equation.

unknown × 1 = 0.133 × 100

unknown = 13.3 mg = **13.3 mg%**

c) To convert from mg/L to mg/dl recall that a deciliter is 100 ml (See Appendix G) and then set up your ratio as in b):

$$\frac{0.133 \text{ mg}}{1 \text{ ml}} = \frac{\text{unknown mg}}{100 \text{ ml}}$$

Cross multiply to solve the equation.

unknown × 1 = 0.133 × 100

unknown = **13.3 mg/dl**

d) To convert 133 mg/L to ppm, proceed as before, using common units. Since ppm can be defined as $g/10^6$ ml, begin by converting the numerator from milligrams to grams using the fact that 1 g = 1000 mg.

$$\frac{133 \, \cancel{mg}}{1 \, L} \times \frac{1 \, g}{1000 \, \cancel{mg}} = \frac{0.133 \, g}{L}$$

Next convert the denominator from liters to milliliters using the fact that 1 L = 1000 ml:

$$\frac{0.133 \, g}{1 \, \cancel{L}} \times \frac{1 \, \cancel{L}}{1000 \, ml} = \frac{0.133 \, g}{1000 \, ml} = 0.000133 \, g \, / \, ml$$

Parts per million (ppm) is here defined as grams per 10^6 milliliters. Therefore, ppm can be determined by using a ratio:

$$\frac{0.133 \, g}{1000 \, ml} = \frac{unknown \, mg}{1,000,000 \, ml}$$

Cross multiply to solve the equation.

unknown × 1000 = 0.133 × 1,000,000

$$unknown = \frac{0.133 \times 1,000,000}{1000}$$

unknown = 133 mg/ml

Therefore, 133 mg/ml = **133 ppm**

e) The last step in this problem is to convert mg/L to mcg/ml. The secret in each of these conversions is to remember to use common units. Convert the numerator from milligrams to micrograms:

$$\frac{133 \ \cancel{mg}}{1 \ L} \times \frac{1000 \ mcg}{1 \ \cancel{mg}} = \frac{133,000 \ mcg}{L}$$

Next convert the denominator from liters to milligrams:

$$\frac{133,000 \ mcg}{1 \ \cancel{L}} \times \frac{1 \ \cancel{L}}{1000 \ ml} = \frac{133 \ mcg}{ml} = 133 \ mcg \ / \ ml$$

It does not matter in which order we convert to common units. You can convert the denominator first if you wish, or do it all in one equation!

$$\frac{133 \ \cancel{mg}}{1 \ \cancel{L}} \times \frac{1000 \ mcg}{1 \ \cancel{mg}} \times \frac{1 \ \cancel{L}}{1000 \ ml} = 133 \ mcg \ / \ ml$$

★ **Example:** *A 10 kg dog is presented to the clinic after ingesting an unknown quantity of alcohol at the owner's Superbowl party. If the beer contains 3.2% ethanol, how much beer has the animal ingested if its blood alcohol level is 0.1 g/dl? (The specific gravity of ethanol is 0.79 g/ml and its volume of distribution is estimated at 0.5 L/kg.)*

Step 1:
Convert the blood alcohol level from g/dl to g/L (See Appendix G):

$$blood \ level \ (g \ / \ L) = \frac{0.1 \ g}{1 \ \cancel{dl}} \times \frac{10 \ \cancel{dl}}{1 \ L} = 1 \ g \ / \ L$$

Step 2:
blood level (g/L) =

$$\frac{amt \ ingested \ (ml) \times (\% \ sol'n \ / \ 100) \times specific \ gravity \ (g \ / \ ml)}{Vd \ (L \ / \ kg) \times wt \ (kg)}$$

Vd = volume of distribution of the substance

Fill in the known quantities and solve for amount ingested:

$$1 \text{ g} / \text{L} = \frac{\text{amt ingested} \times (3.2 / 100) \times 0.79 \text{ g} / \text{ml}}{0.5 \text{ L} / \text{kg} \times 10 \text{ kg}}$$

$$\frac{1 \text{ g}}{\text{L}} = \frac{\text{amt ingested} \times 0.02528 \text{ g} / \text{ml}}{5 \text{ L}}$$

Cross multiply to solve the equation:

$$5 = \text{amt ingested} \times 0.02528 \text{ g}$$

$$\text{amt ingested} = \frac{5}{0.02528 \text{ g}}$$

amt ingested = 0.19778 g ≈ **6.6 oz** (See Appendix G for conversions from g to oz.)

★ **Example:** *One study of a veterinary product containing both DEET (9%) and fenvalerate (0.09%) determined that applying more than 0.7 oz/kg of body weight could cause fatalities in cats. Self-grooming after topical application of the pesticide was 50–150 times more likely to cause toxicity.*

a) How much of the 7 oz can be used on a 5 kg cat if the maximum level is 0.7 oz/kg of body weight?

oz to apply = wt (kg) × 0.7 oz/kg

oz to apply = 5 kg × 0.7 oz/kg

oz to apply = 3.5 oz

$$\frac{3.5 \text{ oz}}{7.0 \text{ oz}} = 0.5 = 50\% \text{ of can}$$

b) How many grams of DEET would a 5 kg cat be exposed to if 3.5 oz of the product (0.7 oz/kg body weight) was applied?

Since the volume of the can was provided in ounces, it should be converted to milliliters first (See Appendix G):

$$ml = \frac{3.5 \text{ oz}}{1} \times \frac{29.57 \text{ ml*}}{1 \text{ oz}}$$

1 oz is often approximated at 30 ml.

$$ml = \frac{3.5 \text{ oz}}{1} \times \frac{30 \text{ ml}}{1 \text{ oz}} = 105 \text{ ml}$$

By definition, $9\% = \dfrac{9 \text{ g}}{100 \text{ ml}}$

$$\frac{9 \text{ g}}{100 \text{ ml}} = \frac{\text{unknown g}}{105 \text{ ml}}$$

Cross multiply to solve the equation.

unknown g × 100 ml = 9 g × 105 ml

$$\text{unknown g} = \frac{9 \text{ g} \times 105}{100}$$

unknown g = **9.45 g**

Or these 2 equations could be combined into one as follows:

unknown g = 9% × 3.5 oz × 30* ml/oz

$$\text{unknown g} = \frac{9 \text{ g}}{100 \text{ ml}} \times \frac{3.5 \text{ oz}}{1} \times \frac{30 \text{ ml}}{1 \text{ oz}}$$

$$\text{unknown g} = \frac{9 \times 3.5 \times 30}{100}$$

unknown g = **9.45 g**

c) The oral LD_{50} (lethal dose that will kill approximately 50% of a group of animals) for mice and rats exposed to DEET is 2400 mg/kg. Did this cat receive a potentially lethal dose of DEET?

$$\text{g / kg} = \frac{\text{amount applied (g)}}{\text{wt of cat (kg)}}$$

$$\text{g / kg} = \frac{9.45 \text{ g}}{5 \text{ kg}}$$

g/kg = 1.89 g/kg

To convert from g/kg to mg/kg use the fact
1 g = 1000 mg:

$$\frac{1.89 \cancel{g}}{1 \text{ kg}} \times \frac{1000 \text{ mg}}{\cancel{g}/\text{kg}} = 1{,}890 \text{ mg/kg}$$

Alternately, the two equations above can be combined into one:

$$\frac{9.45 \cancel{g}}{5 \text{ kg}} \times \frac{1000 \text{ mg}}{1 \cancel{g}} = 1{,}890 \text{ mg / kg}$$

While the cat was not exposed to an amount of DEET considered toxic for mice and rats, sensitivity to DEET can vary among species. The toxicity of other ingredients, active and inert, should also be considered.

★ **Example:** *A cat is presented with a serum lead level of 1.99 ppm (normal < 0.025 ppm). Convert*

1.99 ppm to a) mg %, b) mg/dl, c) mg/ml, and d) mcg/ml.

a) To convert 1.99 ppm to mg %:

By definition, 1.99 ppm = 1.99 g/1,000,000 ml

Convert to mg:

$$\frac{1.99 \text{ g}}{1,000,000 \text{ ml}} \times \frac{1000 \text{ mg}}{1 \text{ g}} = \frac{1,990 \text{ mg}}{1,000,000 \text{ ml}}$$

To convert to mg % (mg/100 ml) set up a ratio:

By definition, mg % = mg/100 ml

$$\frac{1,990 \text{ mg}}{1,000,000 \text{ ml}} = \frac{\text{unknown mg}}{100 \text{ ml}}$$

Cross multiply to solve the equation.

unknown mg × 1,000,000 = 1,990 × 100

$$\text{unknown mg} = \frac{199,000}{1,000,000}$$

unknown mg = 0.199 mg

Therefore, 1.99 ppm = **0.199 mg%**

b) To convert to mg/dl (mg/100 ml):

By definition, 1.99 ppm = 1.99 g/1,000,000 ml

Convert to mg:

$$\frac{1.99 \text{ g}}{1,000,000 \text{ ml}} \times \frac{1000 \text{ mg}}{1 \text{ g}} = \frac{1,990 \text{ mg}}{1,000,000 \text{ ml}}$$

To convert to mg/dl set up a ratio.

By definition, mg/dl = mg/100 ml

$$\frac{1,990 \text{ mg}}{1,000,000 \text{ ml}} = \frac{\text{unknown mg}}{100 \text{ ml}}$$

Cross multiply to solve the equation:

unknown × 1,000,000 = 1,990 × 100

$$\text{unknown} = \frac{199,000}{1,000,000}$$

unknown = 0.199 mg/dl

Therefore, 1.99 ppm = 0.199 **mg/dl**

c) To convert to mg/ml:

By definition, 1.99 ppm = 1.99 g/1,000,000 ml

Convert to mg:

$$\frac{1.99 \cancel{\text{g}}}{1,000,000 \text{ ml}} \times \frac{1000 \text{ mg}}{1 \cancel{\text{g}}} = \frac{1,990 \text{ mg}}{1,000,000 \text{ ml}}$$

Set up a ratio:

$$\frac{1,990 \text{ mg}}{1,000,000 \text{ ml}} = \frac{\text{unknown mg}}{1 \text{ ml}}$$

Cross multiply to solve the equation:

unknown × 1,000,000 = 1,990 × 1

$$\text{unknown} = \frac{1,990}{1,000,000}$$

unknown = 0.00199 **mg/ml**

Therefore, mg/ml = ppm/1000

d) To convert ppm to mcg/ml:

By definition, 1.99 ppm = 1.99 g/1,000,000 ml

Convert to mg:

$$\frac{1.99 \, \cancel{g}}{1,000,000 \, ml} \times \frac{1000 \, mg}{1 \, \cancel{g}} = \frac{1,990 \, mg}{1,000,000 \, ml}$$

To convert to mcg/ml, use the fact that 1 mg = 1000 mcg:

$$\text{unknown} = \frac{1,990 \, \cancel{mg}}{1,000,000 \, ml} \times \frac{1000 \, mcg}{1 \, \cancel{mg}}$$

$$\text{unknown} = \frac{1,990,000 \, mcg}{1,000,000 \, ml}$$

unknown = 1.99 mcg/ml

This can also be accomplished in a single equation:

$$\frac{1.99 \, \cancel{g}}{1,000,000 \, ml} \times \frac{1000 \, \cancel{mg}}{1 \, \cancel{g}} \times \frac{1000 \, mcg}{1 \, \cancel{mg}} = 1.99 \, mcg \, / \, ml$$

Therefore, 1.99 ppm = **1.99 mcg/ml**

★ **Example**: *A 9 lb cat has ingested Tylenol®. How much of the antidote acetylcysteine is required to treat the cat with a 140 mg/kg loading dose, followed by 20 mg/kg orally every 4 hours for 3 days?*

Step 1:
To determine the loading dose, convert the cat's weight from pounds to kilograms and multiply it by 140 mg/kg:

$$\text{wt (kg)} = \frac{1 \, kg}{2.2 \, lb}$$

$$\text{wt (kg)} = \frac{9 \,\cancel{lb}}{1} \times \frac{1 \text{ kg}}{2.2 \,\cancel{lb}}$$

$$\text{wt (kg)} = 4.09 \text{ kg}$$

$$\text{loading dose} = \frac{140 \text{ mg}}{1 \text{ kg}} \times \text{animal's wt (kg)}$$

$$\frac{140 \text{ mg}}{1 \,\cancel{kg}} \times \frac{4.09 \,\cancel{kg}}{1} = 573 \text{ mg}$$

Step 2:
To calculate the maintenance dose multiply the cat's weight (4.09 kg) by the 20 mg/kg/dose:

$$\text{mg/dose} = \text{maintenance dose} \times \text{animal's wt (kg)}$$

$$\text{dose} = 20 \text{ mg/kg/dose} \times 4.09 \text{ kg}$$

$$\text{dose} = 81.8 \text{ mg}$$

Step 3:
To determine the number of doses per day, divide 24 hours per day by 1 dose/4 hr:

$$\text{doses / day} = \frac{24 \,\cancel{hr}}{1 \text{ day}} \times \frac{1 \text{ dose}}{4 \,\cancel{hr}} = 6 \text{ doses / day}$$

Step 4:
Multiply the number of doses per day by the number of days of maintenance therapy to determine the total number of 81.8 mg maintenance doses that are required:

$$6 \text{ doses/day} \times 3 \text{ days} = 18 \text{ doses}$$

To determine the amount of acetylcysteine required for the maintenance doses, multiply the number of doses by 81.8 mg/dose:

18 doses × 81.8 mg/dose = 1,472.4 mg

Alternate Method:
The amount of acetylcysteine required for maintenance could be determined in one single step by using the equation

drug required for maintenance dosing =
wt (lb) × 1 kg/2.2 lb × maintenance dose (mg/kg) × duration of therapy (days) × 24 hours/day × dosing frequency (e.g., 1 dose/unknown hr)

$$\text{dose} = \frac{\text{wt (lb)}}{1} \times \frac{1\ \text{kg}}{2.2\ \text{lb}} \times \frac{20\ \text{mg/kg}}{1\ \text{dose}} \times \frac{3\ \text{days}}{1} \times \frac{24\ \text{hr}}{1\ \text{day}} \times \frac{1\ \text{dose}}{4\ \text{hr}}$$

$$\text{dose} = \frac{9\ \cancel{\text{lb}}}{1} \times \frac{1\ \cancel{\text{kg}}}{2.2\ \cancel{\text{lb}}} \times \frac{20\ \text{mg}\ /\cancel{\text{kg}}}{1\ \cancel{\text{dose}}} \times \frac{3\ \cancel{\text{days}}}{1} \times \frac{6\ \cancel{\text{doses}}}{1\ \cancel{\text{day}}}$$

dose = 1,472.7 mg

Step 5:
To determine the total amount of acetylcysteine required to treat this 9 lb cat, add the loading dose and maintenance dose together:

total medication required = loading dose + maintenance dose

total medication = 573 mg + 1472.7 mg

total medication = 2,045.7 mg

Step 6:
Acetylcysteine comes as a 10% solution. How many milliliters are needed to provide 2,045.7 mg? Remember that by definition,
10% = 10 g/100 ml = 100 mg/ml.

Divide the total dose by the concentration of the solution, making sure to use like units in the numerator and denominator:

$$\text{volume required (ml)} = \frac{\text{total dose (mg)}}{\text{concentration (mg / ml)}}$$

$$\text{volume} = \frac{2,045.7 \text{ mg}}{100 \text{ mg / ml}}$$

volume = 10.457 ml

volume ≈ **10.5 ml**

★ **Example:** *A 40 lb dog is presented with ethylene glycol toxicity. Since the antidote, 4-methylpyrazole (4-MP), is unavailable you decide to use ethanol as an antidote. Ethanol is used to treat ethylene glycol toxicity in dogs at a dose of 5.5 ml of 20% ethanol per kilogram of body weight every 4 hours for 5 doses, then daily for 5 days. How much absolute (100%) alcohol is needed to treat this 40 lb dog?*

Step 1:
Convert the weight of the dog from pounds to kilograms using the equation:

$$\text{wt (kg)} = \text{wt (lb)} \times \frac{1 \text{ kg}}{2.2 \text{ lb}}$$

$$wt \ (kg) = \frac{40 \ \text{lb}}{1} \times \frac{1 \ kg}{2.2 \ \text{lb}}$$

wt (kg) = 18.2 kg

Step 2:
A dose of 5.5 ml of 20% ethanol per kilogram of animal weight is required. To calculate the amount of 20% alcohol required per dose, multiply the dog's weight in kilograms by 5.5 ml/kg/dose:

vol of 20% ethanol required = wt (kg) × dose (ml/kg)

vol = 18.2 kg × 5.5 ml of 20% alcohol/kg/dose

volume = 100.1 ml of 20% alcohol

Step 3:
Absolute alcohol is 100% alcohol. To calculate the amount of absolute or 100% alcohol required per dose use the equation:

strength × quantity = strength × quantity

100.1 ml × 20% = 100% × unknown ml

$$unknown \ ml = \frac{100.1 \ ml \times 20\%}{100\%}$$

unknown ml = 20.02 ml

Step 4:
To calculate the amount of absolute alcohol needed for the entire treatment, determine the number of doses required and multiply by the amount required per dose:

$$\text{total volume required} = \frac{\text{volume}}{\text{dose}} \times \text{doses}$$

$$\text{total volume} = \frac{20.02 \text{ ml}}{1 \text{ dose}} \times \frac{10 \text{ doses}}{1}$$

total volume = 200.2 ml

★ **Example:** *A 6 lb cat is accidently dipped in malathion. After a bath, it is decided that medical treatment should be initiated. Atropine is given in conjunction with pralidoxime at a dose of 0.05 mg/kg to treat organophosphate toxicity. How many milliliters of atropine should be used per dose as a antidote?*

Step 1:
Convert to common units by converting the cat's weight from pounds to kilograms:

$$\text{wt (kg)} = \text{wt (lb)} \times \frac{1 \text{ kg}}{2.2 \text{ lb}}$$

$$\text{wt (kg)} = \frac{6 \text{ lb}}{1} \times \frac{1 \text{ kg}}{2.2 \text{ lb}}$$

wt (kg) = 2.7 kg

Step 2:
Determine the amount of atropine required, in milligrams, by multiplying the dose required (mg/kg) by the weight of the animal (kg):

specific dose required = dose (mg/kg) × wt (kg)

dose = 0.05 mg/kg × 2.7 kg

dose = 0.135 mg

Step 3:

Since atropine is available as a 1/120 grain per milliliter solution, its concentration must first be determined in mg/ml, rather than in grains/ml, so you can calculate how many milliliters are required to deliver 0.135 mg. Convert the strength of the atropine from grains to milligrams by multiplying by the conversion factor 64.8 mg = 1 grain (See Appendix G):

$$\text{concentration (mg / ml)} = \frac{1 \,\cancel{\text{grain}}}{1 \text{ ml}} \times \frac{64.8 \text{ mg}}{1 \,\cancel{\text{grain}}}$$

$$\text{concentration} = \frac{\dfrac{1}{120} \,\cancel{\text{grain}}}{\text{ml}} \times \frac{64.8 \text{ mg}}{1 \,\cancel{\text{grain}}}$$

$$\text{concentration} = \frac{\dfrac{64.8 \text{ mg}}{120}}{1}$$

concentration = 0.54 mg/ml

Step 4:

Divide the dose required (mg) by the concentration of atropine (mg/ml) to determine the volume of atropine required:

$$\text{volume dose (ml)} = \frac{\text{dose (mg)}}{\text{concentration (mg/ml)}}$$

$$\text{volume dose (ml)} = \frac{0.135 \text{ mg}}{0.54 \text{ mg/ml}}$$

volume dose = **0.25 ml of 1/120 grain atropine**

★ **Example:** *Calcium-EDTA is used to treat lead toxicity in a variety of species including birds. If a 90 g cockatiel is suffering from lead toxicity and the recommended dose of Ca-EDTA is*

10 mg/kg IM every 8 hours, how much of a 6.6% solution of Ca-EDTA is required per treatment?

Step 1:
Convert the bird's weight from grams to kilograms by multiplying by the conversion factor 1 kg =1000 g (See Appendix G):

$$wt\ (kg) = wt\ (g) \times \frac{1\ kg}{1000\ g}$$

$$wt\ (kg) = \frac{90\ \cancel{g}}{1} \times \frac{1\ kg}{1000\ \cancel{g}}$$

$$wt\ (kg) = 0.09\ kg$$

Step 2:
To determine the number of milligrams of Ca-EDTA required per dose, multiply the weight of the bird in kilograms by the dose (10 mg/kg):

$$dose = \frac{0.09\ \cancel{kg}}{1} \times \frac{10\ mg}{1\ \cancel{kg}}$$

$$dose = 0.9\ mg$$

Alternate Method:
Steps 1 and 2 could be combined into one step:

$$dose = wt\ (g) \times \frac{1\ kg}{1000\ g} \times \frac{10\ mg}{1\ kg}$$

$$dose = \frac{90\ \cancel{g}}{1} \times \frac{1\ \cancel{kg}}{1000\ \cancel{g}} \times \frac{10\ mg}{1\ \cancel{kg}}$$

$$dose = 0.9\ mg$$

Step 3:
To determine the amount of 6.6% (by definition, 6.6% = 6.6 g/100 ml) solution that will be required per treatment, convert to common units:

$$\text{ml / dose} = \frac{\text{mg required / dose} \times 1 \text{ g / } 1000 \text{ mg}}{\text{concentration (g / } 100 \text{ ml)}}$$

$$\text{ml / dose} = \frac{0.9 \text{ mg / dose} \times 1 \text{ g / } 1000 \text{ mg}}{6.6 \text{ g / } 100 \text{ ml}}$$

$$\text{ml/dose} = \frac{0.9 \times 0.001}{0.066 \text{ ml}}$$

dose = **0.014 ml**

Alternate Method:
The concentration of the 6.6% Ca-EDTA could be converted from 6.6 g/100 ml to mg/ml:

conc (mg) = conc (g/100 ml) × 1000 mg/ g

$$\text{conc} = \frac{6.6 \text{ g}}{100 \text{ ml}} \times \frac{1000 \text{ mg}}{1 \text{ g}}$$

$$\text{conc} = \frac{6,600 \text{ mg}}{100 \text{ ml}}$$

conc (mg) = 66 mg/ml

The volume required can then be determined by dividing the dose in milligrams by the concentration in milligrams per milliliter:

$$\text{volume} = \frac{0.9 \text{ mg/dose}}{66 \text{ mg/ml}}$$

volume = **0.014 ml**

★ **Example:** *4-Methylparazole (4-MP) can be used to treat ethylene glycol toxicity in dogs. (It does not appear to be effective in cats.) A protocol of 20 mg/kg I.V. initially, followed by 15 mg/kg at 12 and 24 hours, and 5 mg/kg at 36 hours is suggested. How much of a 5% solution is required to treat a 40 lb dog?*

Step 1:
Convert the dog's weight from pounds to kilograms
(See Appendix G):

$$wt \ (kg) = wt \ (lb) \times \frac{1 \ kg}{2.2 \ lb}$$

$$wt \ (kg) = 40 \ lb \times \frac{1 \ kg}{2.2 \ lb}$$

$$wt = 18.2 \ kg$$

Step 2:
Calculate the initial dose required:

initial dose = dose (mg/kg) × wt (kg)

initial dose = 20 mg/kg × 18.2 kg

initial dose = 364 mg

Step 3:
Calculate the dose required at 12 and 24 hours:

mg/dose = dose (mg/kg) × wt (kg)

mg/dose = 15 mg/kg × 18.2 kg

mg/dose = 273 mg/dose

Step 4:
Calculate the dose required at 36 hours:

dose = dose (mg/kg) × wt (kg)

dose = 5 mg/kg × 18.2 kg

dose = 91 mg

Step 5:
Determine the total amount of 4-MP required:

total dose =
initial dose + 12 hr dose + 24 hr dose + 36 hr dose

total dose = 364 mg + (2 × 273 mg) + 91 mg

total dose = 1,001 mg

Step 6:
To determine the amount of 5% solution that will be required, convert 5% to mg/ml:

By definition, $5\% = \dfrac{5\text{ g}}{100\text{ ml}}$

$5\% = \dfrac{5\text{ g}}{100\text{ ml}} \times \dfrac{1000\text{ mg}}{\text{g}}$

$5\% = \dfrac{5{,}000\text{ mg}}{100\text{ ml}}$

$5\% = \dfrac{50\text{ mg}}{\text{ml}}$

Step 7:
Divide the amount required (mg) by the concentration available (mg/ml) to determine the volume required:

$\text{volume required} = \dfrac{\text{dose (mg)}}{\text{concentration (mg / ml)}}$

$\text{volume} = \dfrac{1{,}001\text{ mg}}{50\text{ mg} / \text{ml}}$

volume = **20.02 ml**

★ **Example:** *Yohimbine has been used to reverse the effects of xylazine in white-tailed deer at a dose of 0.125 mg/kg. If a buck weighs 150 lb, how many milliliters of yohimbine are needed?*

Step 1:
Convert the weight of the deer from pounds to kilograms:

$$\text{wt (kg)} = \text{wt (lb)} \times \frac{1 \text{ kg}}{2.2 \text{ lb}}$$

$$\text{wt (kg)} = 150 \text{ lb} \times \frac{1 \text{ kg}}{2.2 \text{ lb}}$$

wt (kg) = 68 kg

Step 2:
Multiply the dose required in mg/kg by the weight of the buck in kilograms:

dose = 0.125 mg/kg × 68 kg

dose = 8.5 mg

Step 3:
Divide the amount of yohimbine required in mg by the concentration in mg/ml:

volume dose = 8.5 mg/(2 mg/ml)

volume dose = **4.25 ml**

★ **Example:** *A client calls you after another veterinarian has prescribed the use of Ovitrol Plus® topically every 48 hours for fleas. The client applied the medication every other day for 12 days at which time the dog developed diarrhea. The*

*referring veterinarian prescribed Peptobismol®
1 Tbs PO q12h. The dog began to seizure and
died two days later. The client estimates that she
used three-quarters of the 16 fluid ounce bottle
over the 12 days and wants to know if her treatment with Ovitrol Plus® killed the dog. The dog
was a 60 lb, 11-year-old Labrador cross with
no history of previous problems.*

The label states that Ovitrol Plus® contains:

methoprene	0.25%
pyrethrin	0.18%
piperonyl butoxide	0.36%
N-octyl bicycloheptene dicarboximide	0.6%
inert ingredients	98.61%

Based on the LD_{50} levels for methoprene, pyrethrin,
pipronyl butoxide, and N-octyl bicycloheptene
dicarboximide, could this animal have developed
lethal toxicity?

Step 1:
Determine the amount of Ovitrol Plus® that was
applied.

amt applied = 3/4 bottle × 16 fl oz × 30 ml/fl oz

amt applied = 360 ml

Step 2:
Determine the amount of methoprene the dog has
been exposed to by multiplying the volume applied
by the concentration of the methoprene:

exposure dose = % × volume
exposure dose = 0.25% × 360 ml

exposure level = (0.25 g/100 ml) × 360 ml
exposure level = 0.9 g

Step 3:
Convert the amount of methoprene applied from grams to milligrams using the fact that 1 gram = 1000 milligrams (See Appendix G):

mg = grams × (1000 mg/g)
mg = 0.9 g × (1000 mg/g)
mg = 900 mg

Step 4:
Convert the dog's weight from pounds to kilograms using the fact that 1 kilogram = 2.2 pounds (See Appendix G):

$$\text{wt (kg)} = \text{wt (lb)} \times \frac{1\text{ kg}}{2.2\text{ lb}}$$

$$\text{wt (kg)} = 60\,\cancel{\text{lb}} \times \frac{1\text{ kg}}{2.2\,\cancel{\text{lb}}}$$

wt = 27.27 kg

Step 5:
Divide the amount of active ingredients applied (in milligrams) by the dog's weight (in kg) to determine the mg/kg exposure level:

$$\text{exposure level} = \frac{\text{amount of active ingredient (mg)}}{\text{animal's weight (kg)}}$$

$$\text{exposure level} = \frac{900\text{ mg}}{27.27\text{ kg}}$$

exposure level = **33 mg/kg**

Conclusion for Methoprene:
Methoprene has an oral LD_{50} in dogs of 5,000 mg/kg. Ovitrol Plus® is a topical preparation. Dermal exposure is usually less toxic than oral ingestion resulting in higher LD_{50} for topical administration. Since the exposure level of methoprene was significantly less (33 mg/kg) than the oral LD_{50} of methoprene (5,000 mg/kg), it is unlikely that the methoprene caused a toxicity.

Step 6:
Determine the amount of pyrethrin the dog has been exposed to by multiplying the volume applied by the concentration of the pyrethrin:

exposure dose = % × volume

Convert % to g/100ml:
exposure dose = (g/100 ml) × volume

$$\text{exposure dose} = \frac{0.18g}{100ml} \times 360 \text{ ml}$$

exposure dose = 0.648 g

Step 7:
Convert the amount of pyrethrin applied from grams to milligrams using the fact that 1 gram = 1000 milligrams (See Appendix G):

mg = grams × (1000 mg/g)
mg = 0.648 g × (1000 mg/g)
mg = 648 mg

Step 8:
Convert the dog's weight from pounds to kilograms using the fact that 1 kilogram = 2.2 pounds (See Appendix G):

$$wt\ (kg) = wt\ (lb) \times \frac{1\ kg}{2.2\ lb}$$

$$wt\ (kg) = 60\ \cancel{lb} \times \frac{1\ kg}{2.2\ \cancel{lb}}$$

wt = 27.27 kg

Step 9:
Divide the amount of active ingredients applied (mg) by the dog's weight (kg) to determine the mg/kg exposure level:

$$exposure\ level = \frac{amount\ of\ active\ ingredient\ (mg)}{animal's\ weight\ (kg)}$$

$$exposure\ level = \frac{648\ mg}{27.27\ kg}$$

exposure level = **23.8 mg/kg**

Conclusion for Pyrethrin:
While pyrethrin LD_{50} levels vary among the oral species, the oral LD_{50} for rats is commonly used. LD_{50} for rats is 2–16 g/kg or 2,000–16,000 mg per kilogram of body weight. Since this dog was exposed to only 23.8 mg/kg, it is unlikely that pyrethrin caused a toxic reaction.

Step 10:
Determine the amount of piperonyl butoxide the dog has been exposed to by multiplying the volume applied by the concentration of the piperonyl butoxide:

exposure dose = % × volume

Convert % to grams per 100 milliliters.

$$exposure\ dose = \frac{g}{100\ ml} \times volume$$

$$\text{exposure dose} = \frac{0.36\ g}{100\ \cancel{ml}} \times 360\ \cancel{ml}$$

exposure dose = 1.3 g

Step 11:

Convert the amount of piperonyl butoxide applied from grams to milligrams using the fact that 1 gram = 1000 milligrams (See Appendix G):

mg = grams × (1000 mg/g)
mg = 1.3 g × (1000 mg/g)
mg = 1,300 mg

Step 12:

As calculated in Step 8:

$$\text{wt (kg)} = \text{wt (lb)} \times \frac{1\ kg}{2.2\ lb}$$

$$\text{wt (kg)} = 60\ \cancel{lb} \times \frac{1\ kg}{2.2\ \cancel{lb}}$$

wt (kg) = 27.27 kg

Step 13:

Divide the amount of active ingredients applied (in milligrams) by the dog's weight (in kg) to determine the mg/kg exposure level:

$$\text{exposure level} = \frac{\text{amount of active ingredient (mg)}}{\text{animal's weight (kg)}}$$

$$\text{exposure level} = \frac{1,300\ mg}{27.27\ kg}$$

exposure level = **47.7 mg/kg**

Conclusion for Piperonyl Butoxide:
The LD_{50} of oral piperonyl butoxide is approximately 7,500 mg/kg, suggesting that the piperonyl butoxide was probably not toxic.

Step 14:
Like piperonyl butoxide, N-octyl bicycloheptene dicarboximide is an insecticide synergist. Although a specific LD_{50} level for N-octyl bicycloheptene dicarboximide is not given, it is believed to be slightly more toxic than piperonyl butoxide. Large doses can cause CNS stimulation followed by depression.

Determine the amount of N-octyl bicycloheptene dicarboximide the dog has been exposed to by multiplying the volume applied by the concentration of the N-octyl bicycloheptene dicarboximide:

exposure dose = % × volume

Convert percent to grams per 100 milliliters.

$$\text{exposure dose} = \frac{0.6 \text{ g}}{100 \text{ ml}} \times 360 \text{ ml}$$

exposure dose = 2.16 g

Step 15:
Convert the amount of N-octyl bicycloheptene dicarboximide applied from grams to milligrams using the fact that 1 gram = 1000 mg (See Appendix G):

mg = grams × (1000 mg/g)
mg = 2.16 g × (1000 mg/g)
mg = 2,160 mg

Step 16:

Convert the dog's weight from pounds to kilograms using the fact that 1 kg = 2.2 lb (See Appendix G):

$$wt \ (kg) = wt \ (lb) \times \frac{1 \ kg}{2.2 \ lb}$$

$$wt \ (kg) = 60 \ \cancel{lb} \times \frac{1 \ kg}{2.2 \ \cancel{lb}}$$

$$wt = 27.27 \ kg$$

Step 17:

Divide the amount of active ingredients applied (mg) by the dog's weight (kg) to determine the mg/kg exposure level:

$$exposure \ level = \frac{amount \ of \ active \ ingredient \ (mg)}{animal's \ weight \ (kg)}$$

$$exposure \ level = \frac{2,160 \ mg}{27.27 \ kg}$$

exposure level = **79.2 mg/kg**

Conclusion for Bicycloheptene:
Although LD_{50} levels vary among species and depend on the route of exposure, it is suggested that none of the chemicals in this formulation were used at levels high enough to be toxic.

★ **Example:** *A 7 lb cat is presented to the clinic with depression, anorexia, and a lead level of 1.99 ppm (normal is < 0.025 ppm). To initiate Ca-EDTA at 50 mg/kg/day, how much 6.6% Ca-EDTA solution is required?*

Step 1:
Convert the weight of the cat from pounds to kilograms (See Appendix G):

$$\text{wt (kg)} = \text{wt (lb)} \times \frac{1 \text{ kg}}{2.2 \text{ lb}}$$

$$\text{wt (kg)} = 7 \,\cancel{\text{lb}} \times \frac{1 \text{ kg}}{2.2 \,\cancel{\text{lb}}}$$

$$\text{wt} = 3.18 \text{ kg}$$

Step 2:
Multiply the dose per day of Ca-EDTA by the weight of the cat in kilograms:

$$\text{dose} = \text{wt (kg)} \times \text{dose}\left(\frac{\text{mg}}{\text{kg / day}}\right)$$

$$\text{dose} = 3.18 \,\cancel{\text{kg}} \times \frac{50 \text{ mg}}{\cancel{\text{kg}} / \text{day}}$$

$$\text{dose} = 159 \text{ mg/day}$$

Step 3:
Determine the volume of 6.6% solution required:

By definition,

$$6.6\% = \frac{6.6 \text{ g}}{100 \text{ ml}} = \frac{66 \text{ mg}}{\text{ml}}$$

$$\text{ml of solution required} = \frac{\text{dose required (mg / day)}}{\text{conc of solution (mg / ml)}}$$

$$\text{volume} = \frac{159 \,\cancel{\text{mg}} / \text{day}}{66 \,\cancel{\text{mg}} / \text{ml}}$$

$$\textbf{volume} = \textbf{2.41 ml/day}$$

★ **Example:** *Clients call you because their 35 lb dog has ingested an entire package of medium Heartgard® tablets. The package contains six doses. Is this quantity of Heartgard® toxic and should you advise the client to induce vomiting?*

Step 1:
A medium size Heartgard® tablet contains 136 mcg of ivermectin. To determine if the amount ingested is toxic, first calculate the total amount ingested by multiplying the concentration per tablet by the number of tablets ingested:

amount ingested (mg) = conc / tablet (mg) × tablets ingested
amount ingested = 136 mcg/tablet × 6 tablets
amount ingested = 816 mcg

Most dogs, with the exception of collies, can receive 200 mcg/kg orally as a single dose without complications. Collies may experience problems at doses above 50 mcg/kg. Determine if this dog has consumed a toxic level of ivermectin.

Step 2:
Convert the dog's weight from pounds to kilograms:

$$\text{wt (kg)} = \text{wt (lb)} \times \frac{1 \text{ kg}}{2.2 \text{ lb}}$$

$$\text{wt (kg)} = 35 \text{ lb} \times \frac{1 \text{ kg}}{2.2 \text{ lb}}$$

wt = 15.9 kg

Step 3:
Then divide the amount ingested (mg) by the weight of the dog (kg):

$$\text{level ingested} = \frac{\text{total dose ingested (mcg)}}{\text{wt (kg)}}$$

$$\text{level ingested} = \frac{816 \text{ mcg}}{15.9 \text{ kg}}$$

level ingested = **51.3 mcg/kg**

As long as the dog is not a collie, it is unlikely that the ingestion of 51.3 mcg/kg of ivermectin will cause toxicity. If treatment is initiated, it is usually supportive. Yohimbine was once suggested to be antidotal but has not proved effective. Picrotoxine has also been suggested, but due to its toxicity, it is not typically used.

★ **Example:** *A dog is presented to your clinic after eating part of an amitraz collar. The toxocologist estimates that the dog has ingested 10 mg of amitraz/kg of body weight and advises you to give 1.5 ml/kg syrup of ipecac to induce vomiting and 0.1 mg/kg of yohimbine as an antidote. If the dog weighs 66 lb, calculate a) the amount of amitraz ingested, b) the dose of yohimbine, c) the dose of syrup of ipecac that should be administered, and d) the dose of atropine.*

a) To calculate the amount of amitraz ingested, first convert the weight of the dog from pounds to kilograms:

$$\text{wt (kg)} = \text{wt (lb)} \times \frac{1 \text{ kg}}{2.2 \text{ lb}}$$

$$\text{wt (kg)} = 66 \cancel{\text{ lb}} \times \frac{1 \text{ kg}}{2.2 \cancel{\text{ lb}}}$$

wt (kg) = 30 kg

Multiply the dog's weight in kilograms by the amount of amitraz ingested in milligrams.

mg ingested = weight × dose (mg/kg)
mg ingested = 30 kg × (10 mg amitraz/kg)
mg ingested = **300 mg amitraz**

b) Calculate the amount of syrup of ipecac to be administered by multiplying the weight of the dog in kilograms by the dose in ml/kg:

vol required (ml) = dosage (ml/kg) × animal's wt (kg)
volume = 1.5 ml/kg × 30 kg
volume = **45 ml**

c) Calculate the amount of yohimbine to be administered by multiplying the dose in mg/kg by the weight of the dog in kilograms:

yohimbine required (mg) = dose (mg/kg) × wt (kg)
dose = 0.1 mg/kg × 30 kg
dose = **3 mg**

Yohimbine is available as a 2 mg/ml solution. To find how much should be administered:

$$\text{volume required (ml)} = \frac{\text{dose (mg)}}{\text{conc (mg / ml)}}$$

$$\text{volume} = \frac{3 \text{ mg}}{2 \text{ mg / ml}}$$

volume = **1.5 ml**

d) Atropine has been used at a dose of 0.02 mg/kg to reverse the bradycardia sometimes associated with amitraz toxicity. What dose of atropine should this animal receive?

atropine required (mg) = dose (mg/kg) × wt (kg)

atropine required = 0.02 mg/kg × 30 kg

atropine required = 6 mg

Atropine is available as a 1/120 grain/ml solution. How much would be needed?

$$\text{volume required (ml)} = \frac{\text{dose (mg)}}{\text{conc (mg / ml)}}$$

The concentration of the solution is given in grains per milliliter, so it must first be converted to milligrams per milliliter:

conc (mg/ml) = conc (grains/ml) × 64.8 mg/grain

conc (mg/ml) = 1/120 grain × 64.8 mg/grain

conc (mg/ml) = 0.54 mg/ml

$$\text{volume required (ml)} = \frac{\text{dose (mg)}}{\text{conc (mg / ml)}}$$

$$\text{volume} = \frac{6 \text{ mg}}{0.54 \text{ mg / ml}}$$

volume = **11.1 ml**

Practice Problems
(See Appendix H for answer)

146. How much yohimbine should be administered to a 600 lb Brahma cross that has received xylazine if the recommended dose is 0.125 mg/kg I.V.? (Xylazine is not commonly used for Brahmas due to sudden death.)

147. How much Narcan® should be administered to a 1,200 lb horse at a dose of 0.01–0.022 mg/kg in order to reverse the excitatory effects of a narcotic?

148. How much of a 0.15% pyrethrin spray would have to be applied to a 120 g hamster to reach the potentially lethal dose (LD_{50}) of 4,000 mg/kg?

149. How much 6.6% Ca-EDTA is required to treat a 15 lb Canada goose at a dose of 10 mg/kg?

150. How much syrup of ipecac would be required to induce emesis in a 7 lb dog if the dosage range is 1–2 ml/kg?

151. How many 6 mg apomorphine tablets are required to induce emesis in a 3 kg Pomeranian at a dose of 0.25 mg/kg?

Equations

Body Surface Area

$$\text{body surface area } (m^2) = \frac{K* \times (\text{wt in g})^{0.67}}{10{,}000}$$

K for dogs and cats = 10.1

concentration × volume = concentration × volume

$$\text{drug dose} = \text{BSA } (m^2) \times \frac{\text{drug dose } (mg)}{m^2}$$

Converting Gallons to Pounds

wt(lb) = specific gravity of liquid × 8.33* × gallons

$$\text{volume (gallons)} = \frac{\text{pounds}}{(\text{specific gravity} \times 8.33*)}$$

1 gallon of water = 8.33 lb

Drug Dosing

$$\text{dose } (mg/ml) = \frac{\text{animal's wt } (g) \times \text{dose } (mg) \times 1000\,mg/g}{\text{concentration of drug } (mg/ml)}$$

$$\text{dose } (ml/kg) = \frac{\text{dose } (mg/kg)}{\text{concentration of drug } (mg/ml)}$$

$$\frac{ml \text{ needed}}{\text{dose required } (mEq)} = \frac{ml \text{ of drug in solution}}{mEq \text{ of drug in solution}}$$

mEq/ml = g/ml × mw × 1000 valence

conc required in mEq = conc (mEq/ml) × vol (ml)

$$\text{tablets} = \frac{\text{dose } (mg)}{\text{tablet strength } (mg)}$$

$$mEq = g/mw^* \times 1000 \times valence^{**}$$
$$mEq = mg/mw \times valence$$
$$mEq = mmoles \times valence$$

$mw = molecular\ weight$
**$valence = charge\ of\ the\ particle$*

$$millimoles = \frac{g \times 1000}{mw} = \frac{mg}{mw}$$

$$mOsm = mEq \times particles$$

$$mOsm = \frac{mg}{mw} \times valence \times particles$$

$$Molarity\ (M) = \frac{moles\ of\ solute}{L\ of\ solution}$$

$$M = \frac{mmoles\ of\ solute}{ml\ of\ solution}$$

$$M = \frac{g/mw}{L}$$

$$Normality\ (N) = \frac{g\ equivalents\ solute}{L}$$

$$N = \frac{mEq\ of\ solute}{ml}$$

$$N = \frac{mg/mw \times valence}{ml}$$

$$parts\ per\ million\ (ppm) = \frac{parts\ solute}{million\ parts\ of\ solution}$$

$$1\ ppm = 1\ part/10^6$$
$$1\ ppm = 1\ g/250\ gal$$
$$1\ ppm = 1\ g/35.3\ ft^3$$
$$dose\ (g) = concentration\ (g/ft^3) \times volume\ (ft^3)$$

$$\text{percentage } (\%) \ 5 \ \frac{g}{100\,ml}$$

$$\text{percentage of error } 5 \ \frac{\text{error} \ 3 \ 100\%}{\text{quantity desired}}$$

$$\text{percentage of alcohol } 5 \ \frac{\text{proof strength}}{2}$$

proof strength = percentage of alcohol × 2

$$\text{ratio } 5 \ \frac{\text{amount of drug needed}}{\text{concentration available}} \ 5 \ \frac{\text{unknown volume to give}}{\text{known volume of drug}}$$

$$\text{valence } 5 \ \frac{mEq \ 3 \ mw}{mg} \ 5 \ \frac{mOsm \ 3 \ mw}{mg \ 3 \ \text{particles}}$$

$$\text{ml per hour } 5 \ \frac{\text{volume to be infused } (ml)}{\text{length of infusion } (hr)}$$

$$\text{ml per minute } 5 \ \frac{\text{volume to be infused } (ml)}{\text{length of infusion } (hr) \ 3 \ 60\,min/hr}$$

$$\text{flow rate per hour } 5 \ \text{dose}/hr \ 5 \ \frac{mg \text{ of drug}}{ml \text{ of solution}}$$

$$\text{drip rate } 5 \ \frac{ml \text{ required}}{\text{time}} \ 3 \ \text{drops}/ml$$

$$\text{concentration in } mg/ml \ 5 \ \frac{mg \text{ of drug}}{ml \text{ of I.V. fluids}}$$

drops/minute 5 rate (ml/min) 3 (drops/ml)

dose (mcg/min) 5 dose (mcg/kg/min) 3 wt (kg)

$$\text{volume } (ml) \ 5 \ \frac{\text{dose } (mcg/min)}{\text{concentration } (mcg/ml)}$$

$$\text{rate (ml/min) } 5 \; \frac{\text{(concentration/hour)}}{\text{(concentration/ml)}}$$

$$\text{medication dose/hr } 5 \; \frac{\text{mg of drug 3 flow rate (ml/hr)}}{\text{solution (ml)}}$$

Temperature Conversion Equations

from Fahrenheit to Celsius: $^{\circ}C = (^{\circ}F - 32) \times 5/9$
from Celsius to Fahrenheit: $^{\circ}F = (9/5 \times \, ^{\circ}C) + 32$
from Celsius to Kelvin $^{\circ}K = \, ^{\circ}C + 273$
from Kelvin to Celsius: $^{\circ}C = \, ^{\circ}K - 273$
from Fahrenheit to Kelvin: $^{\circ}K = (^{\circ}F - 32) \times 5/9 + 273$
for Kelvin to Fahrenheit: $^{\circ}F = 9/5 \, (^{\circ}K - 273) + 32$

Volume Equations

triangular trough = $1/2$ base $\times$ height $\times$ length
rectangular trough = length $\times$ width $\times$ height
cylindrical trough = $3.14 \times (\text{radius})^2 \times$ height
truncated cone = $1.05 \times h \times [(r1)^2 + (r1 \times r2) + (r2)^2]$

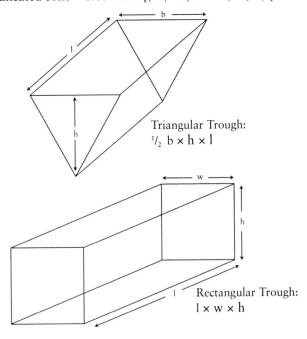

Triangular Trough:
$^{1}/_{2}\ b \times h \times l$

Rectangular Trough:
$l \times w \times h$

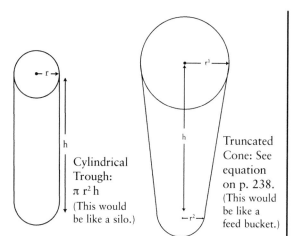

Cylindrical
Trough:
$\pi r^2 h$
(This would
be like a silo.)

Truncated
Cone: See
equation
on p. 238.
(This would
be like a
feed bucket.)

ppm = g/1,000,000 ml = mg/L = mcg/ml

mg% = mg/100 ml

mg/dl = mg/100 ml

mg/ml = (mg%) × 100 = (mg/dl) × 100 = ppm/1000 = g/L

$$\text{doses available} = \frac{\text{strength of the tablet (mg)} \times \text{tablets}}{\text{mg/dose}}$$

$$\text{doses available} = \frac{\text{capsules} \times \text{amt. of AI* per capsule}}{\text{amt. of AI* contained in each dose}}$$

total mg required = mg/dose × doses/day × days

capsules or tablets needed =

$$\frac{\text{total number of mg required}}{\text{mg per commercial capsule or tablet}}$$

$$\frac{\text{single dose}}{\text{total doses}} = \frac{\text{wt of single dose}}{\text{wt of total doses}}$$

diluent required =

$$\frac{total\ amount\ of\ AI^*}{amt.\ of\ AI^*\ per\ dose}\ 3\ wt/dose)\ 2\ wt\ of\ AI^*$$

AI = active ingredient

total mg required = mg/dose × doses/day × days

capsules or tablets needed =

$$\frac{total\ mg\ required}{strength\ of\ one\ capsule\ or\ tablet}$$

$$total\ volume\ required\ 5\ \frac{total\ mg\ required}{concentration\ per\ ml}$$

$$\frac{dose\ desired}{volume\ required}\ 5\ \frac{concentration}{1\ ml}$$

volume × strength = volume × strength

$$ml/vial\ 5\ \frac{concentration\ /vial}{desired\ concentration\ /ml}$$

concentration × volume = concentration × volume

$$ml\ of\ commercial\ prep.\ 5\ \frac{mg\ required}{conc\ commercial\ prep.\ (mg/ml)}$$

Basal Energy Requirements
(BER) = $K^* \times (wt\ in\ kg)^{0.75}$

K is the BER coefficient for various animal types.

a) Mammals K = 70
b) Marsupials K = 49
c) Passerine birds K = 129
d) Nonpasserine birds K = 78
e) Reptiles K = 10

Adjusted Energy Requirements (AER)

a) Enclosure rest = 1 to 1.25 × BER
b) Starvation = 1 to 1.25 × BER
c) Postsurgery = 1.25 × BER
d) Severe burns = 1.5 to 2 × BER
e) Sepsis = 1.5 to 2 × BER
f) Trauma = 1.5 × BER
g) Cancer = 1.5 × BER
h) Hepatic disease = 1.25 × BER
i) Severe renal disease (e.g. BUN > 80) = 1.25 × BER

grams of nitrogen required = AER/Kcal per gram of nitrogen

Kcal required/g nitrogen

a) Enclosure rest   1 g N: 125 to 150 Kcal
b) Nonstress starvation   1 g N: 125 to 150 Kcal
c) Postsurgery   1 g N: 125 Kcal
d) Severe burns   1 g N: 80 to 100 Kcal
e) Sepsis   1 g N: 80 to 125 Kcal
f) Trauma   1 g N: 100 to 125 Kcal
g) Cancer   1 g N: 100 to 125 Kcal
h) Hepatic insufficiency   1 g N: 200 Kcal
i) Severe renal disease   1 g N: 200 to 500 Kcal

$$\text{daily feed requirements } \frac{\text{Kcal required /day}}{\text{caloric content of the diet}}$$

Note: Food calories are referred to as kilocalories (Kcal). Kilocalories are used when determining caloric requirements.

total nonprotein cal =
Kcal provided by lipids + Kcals provided by detrose

$$\text{dextrose solution required} = \frac{\text{Kcal of dextrose needed}}{\text{conc of dextrose (Kcal/ml)}}$$

$$\text{g of nitrogen required } 5 \ \frac{\text{total calories}}{\text{Kcal to N ratio}}$$

g amino acids = g nitrogen × (6.26 g amino acids / 1 g N)

$$\text{AA solution required} = \frac{\text{g of AA needed}}{\text{conc of AA solution (g/100 ml)}}$$

vol of additives =
total vol – vol for calories + vol of proteins

LD_{50} = lethal dose (amount) that will kill approximately 50% of a group of animals

blood level (g/L) =
amt ingested (ml) × (% solution/100) × specific gravity (g/ml) × Vd (L/kg) × wt (kg)

conc (%) × vol (ml) = conc (g/100 ml) × vol (ml)

drug required for maintenance dosing = (animal's wt in lb × 1 kg/2.2 lb) × maintenance dose (mg/kg) × duration of therapy in days × 24 hours/day × dosing frequency (e.g., 1 dose/unknown hr)

$$\text{volume required (ml) } 5 \ \frac{\text{total dose (ml)}}{\text{concentration (mg/ml)}}$$

Abbreviations

AA	amino acids	ft	foot
ac	before meals	ft³	cubic foot
ad	left ear	gal	gallon
AER	adjusted energy requirement	GI	gastrointestinal
AI	active ingredient	g, gm	gram
Al	aluminum	gr	grain
alb	albumin	gtt(s)	drop(s)
AM	morning	H	hydrogen
amp	ampule	HAL	hyperalimentation
amt	amount	HBC	hit by car
as	left ear	hr	hour
au	both ears	hs	bedtime
BER	basal energy requirement	IM	intramuscular
		in., in	inch
bicarb	bicarbonate	IP	intraperitoneal
BID	twice a day	IU	International Units
BSA	body surface area	I.V.	intravenous
BUN	blood urea nitrogen	IVPB	intravenous piggyback
C	carbon	K	potassium
°C	degrees Celsius	°K	degree Kelvin
Ca	calcium	Kcal	kilocalorie
cap	capsule	kg	kilogram
Cl	chlorine	km	kilometer
cm	centimeter	L	liter
cc (ml)	cubic centimeter	lb	pound
cm³	cubic centimeter	LD₅₀	lethal dose that will kill approximately 50% of a group of animals
conc	concentration		
DHT	dihydrotachysterol		
disp	dispense	LR	lactated Ringer's solution
dl	deciliter (100 ml)	LRS	
EFA	essential fatty acid	M	molarity
°F	degrees Fahrenheit	m²	meter squared
Fe	iron	mcg	microgram

ft = foot; ft³ = cubic foot; LD₅₀ rendered below.

LD_{50} lethal dose that will kill approximately 50% of a group of animals

mEq	milliequivalent	q	every
MER	maintenance energy requirement	QD	every day
		QID	four times a day
mg	milligram	qs	a sufficient quantity
Mg	magnesium		
min	minute	qt	quart
ml	milliliter	RL	Ringer's lactate solution
mm	millimole	RLS	
mOsm	milliosmole	RQ	respiratory quotient
4-MP	4-methypyrazole	SC	subcutaneously
mw	molecular weight	Sig	directions to patient
N	nitrogen, normality	sp gr	specific gravity
Na	sodium	stat	immediately
N/A	not applicable	SQ	subcutaneously
NEJM	*New England Journal of Medicine*	sub Q	subcutaneously
		susp	suspension
ng	nanogram	tab	tablet
NS	normal saline	Tbs	tablespoon
O	oxygen	TID	three times a day
od	right eye	TPN	total parenteral nutrition
os	left eye		
ou	each eye	tsp	teaspoon
oz	ounce	tx	treatment
		ut dict	as directed
P	phosphorus	USP	United States Pharmacopeia
pc	after meals		
PM	evening	UUN	urine urea nitrogen
PN	parenteral nutrition	val	valence
PNU	protein nitrogen unit	Vd	volume of distribution
ppm	parts per million		
PPN	partial parenteral nutrition	vit	vitamin
		vol	volume
po, PO	by mouth	v/v	volume/volume
PO$_4$	phosphate	r	radius
prn	as needed	RBC	red blood cell
pt	pint		

RDA	recommended dietary allowance	w/v	weight/volume
wt	weight	w/w	weight/weight
		yr	year

Body Surface Area for Dogs and Cats

Weight in kilograms	Meters squared	Weight in kilograms	Meters squared
0.5	0.06	26	0.92
1.0	0.10	27	0.94
2.0	0.16	28	0.96
3.0	0.22	29	0.99
4.0	0.26	30	1.01
5.0	0.30	31	1.03
6.0	0.34	32	1.05
7.0	0.38	33	1.08
8.0	0.42	34	1.10
9.0	0.45	35	1.12
10.0	0.48	36	1.14
11.0	0.52	37	1.16
12.0	0.55	38	1.18
13.0	0.58	39	1.20
14.0	0.61	40	1.22
15.0	0.63	41	1.24
16.0	0.66	42	1.26
17	0.69	43	1.28
18	0.72	44	1.30
19	0.74	45	1.32
20	0.77	46	1.34
21	0.79	47	1.36
22	0.82	48	1.38
23	0.84	49	1.40
24	0.87	50	1.42
25	0.89		

Appendix

Table of Elements

Name	Symbol	Valence	Atomic Weight
Actinium	Ac	+3	227.0
Aluminum	Al	+3	26.98
Americium	Am	+3,+6	243.0
Antimony	SB	+3,+5	121.7
Argon	Ar	0	39.95
Arsenic	As	+3,+5	74.92
Astatine	At	+1,+5,+7	210.0
Barium	Ba	+2	137.3
Berkelium	Bk	+3,+4	247.0
Beryllium	Be	+2	9.01
Bismuth	Bi	+3,+5	208.98
Boron	B	+3	10.81
Bromine	Br	+1,+5	79.91
Cadmium	Cd	+2	112.4
Calcium	Ca	+2	40.08
Californium	Cf	+3	249.0
Carbon	C	+2,+4	12.01
Cerium	Ce	+3,+4	140.1
Cesium	Cs	+1	132.9
Chlorine	Cl	+1,+5,+7	35.45
Chromium	Cr	+2,+3,+6	51.996
Cobalt	Co	+2,+3	58.93
Copper	Cu	+1,+2	63.54
Curium	Cm	+3	247.0
Dysprosium	Dy	+3	162.5
Einsteinium	Es	+3	254.0
Erbium	Er	+3	167.26
Europium	Eu	+2,+3	151.96
Fermium	Fm	+3	253.0
Fluorine	F	−1	18.998
Francium	Fr	+1	223.0
Gadolinium	Gd	+3	157.25
Gallium	Ga	+3	69.72
Germanium	Ge	+2,+4	72.59

Name	Symbol	Valence	Atomic Weight
Gold	Au	+1,+3	196.96
Hafnium	Hf	+4	178.49
Helium	He	0	4.0
Holmium	Ho	+3	164.93
Hydrogen	H	+1	1.008
Iodine	I	+1,+5,+7	126.90
Indium	In	+3	114.82
Iridium	Ir	+3,+4	192.2
Iron	Fe	+2,+3	55.847
Krypton	Kr	0	83.80
Lanthanum	La	+3	138.91
Lawrencium	Lw	+3	257.0
Lead	Pb	+2,+4	207.19
Lithium	Li	+1	6.939
Lutetium	Lu	+3	174.97
Magnesium	Mg	+2	24.312
Manganese	Mn	+2,3,4,7	54.938
Mendelevium	Md	+2,+3	256.0
Mercury	Hg	+1,+2	200.59
Molybdenum	Mo	+6	95.94
Neodymium	Nd	+3	144.24
Neon	Ne	0	20.18
Neptunium	Np	+3,4,5,6	237.0
Nickel	Ni	+2,+3	58.71
Niobium	Nb	+3,+5	92.91
Nitrogen	N	+1,2,3,+4, +5	14.01
Nobelium	No	+2,+3	253.0
Osmium	Os	+3,+4	190.2
Oxygen	O	–2	15.999
Palladium	Pd	+2,+4	106.4
Phosphorus	P	+3,+5	30.97
Platinum	Pt	+2,+4	195.1
Plutonium	Pu	+3,4,5,6	242.0
Polonium	Po	+2,+4	210.0

Name	Symbol	Valence	Atomic Weight
Potassium	K	−1	39.10
Praseodymium	Pr	+3	140.9
Promethium	Pm	+3	147.0
Protactinium	Pa	+4,+5	231.0
Radium	Ra	+2	225.0
Radon	Rn	0	222.0
Rhenium	Re	+4,6,7	186.2
Rhodium	Rh	+3	102.9
Rubidium	Rb	+1	85.47
Ruthenium	Ru	+3	101.07
Samarium	Sm	+2,+3	150.35
Scandium	Sc	+3	44.956
Selenium	Se	+4,+6,−2	78.96
Silicon	Si	+2,+4	28.086
Silver	Ag	+1	83.80
Sodium	Na	+1	22.99
Strontium	Sr	+2	87.62
Sulfur	S	−2,+4,+6	32.064
Tantalum	Ta	+5	180.95
Technetium	Tc	+4,6,7	99.0
Tellurium	Te	−2,+4,+6	127.6
Terbium	Tb	+3	158.92
Thallium	Tl	+1,+3	204.37
Thorium	Th	+4	232.04
Thulium	Tm	+3	168.93
Tin	Sn	+2,+4	118.69
Titanium	Ti	+2,3,4	47.9
Tungsten	W	+6	183.85
Uranium	U	+3,4,5,6	238.03
Vanadium	V	+2,3,4,5	50.942
Xenon	Xe	0	131.30
Ytterbium	Yb	+2,+3	173.04
Zinc	Zn	+2	65.37
Zirconium	Zr	+4	91.22

Units and Systems of Measure

Metric Measures

Prefix	Symbol	Value	
deci	d	$10^{-1} = 0.1$	one-tenth
centi	c	$10^{-2} = 0.01$	one-hundredth
milli	m	$10^{-3} = 0.001$	one-thousandth
micro	μ	$10^{-6} = 0.000001$	one-millionth
nano	n	10^{-9}	one-billionth
pico	p	10^{-12}	
femto	f	10^{-15}	
atto	a	10^{-18}	
deca/deka	da/dk	$10^{1} = 10$	
hekto	h	$10^{2} = 100$	
kilo	k	$10^{3} = 1000$	
myria	my	$10^{4} = 10,000$	
mega	M	$10^{6} = 1,000,000$	
giga	G	10^{9}	
tera	T	10^{12}	
peta	P	10^{15}	
exa	E	10^{18}	

Volume

Metric

1 ml = 1 cc
     = 0.0610 in.^{3}
1 L = 1000 ml
     = 1 dm^3
     = 0.2642 U.S. gal
     = 0.220 Imp gal
1 m^3 = 1.3080 yd^3

Apothecary

1 ml = 16.23 minims
1 minim = 0.062 ml

Avoirdupois

1 fluid oz = 29.57 ml
1 pt   = 473.2 ml
1 qt   = 946.4 ml
1 gallon = 3,785 ml
1 ft^3 = 0.0283 m^3
1 yd^3 = 27 ft^3
          = 0.7646 m^3
1 bushel = 35.239 L

Weight

Metric

1 mg   = 1000 mcg
1 g   = 1000 mg
1 kg   = 1000 g

Apothecary

1 grain = 64.8 mg
1 mg   = 1/65 grain
1 g   = 15.54 grain
1 oz   = 31.1 g

Avoirdupois

1 oz   = 28.35 g
         = 437.5 gr
1 lb   = 16 oz
         = 454 g
1 kg   = 2.2 lb

Lenth

1 mm	= 0.0394 in.
1 cm	= 10 mm = 0.3937 in.
1 meter (m)	= 100 cm = 1.0936 yd
1 kilometer (km)	= 1000 m = 0.6214 mile
1 inch	= 25.4 mm
1 ft	= 0.3048 m
1 yard	= 0.9144 m
1 mile	= 1.6094 km

Area

1 cm^2	= 0.155 in.^{2}
1 m^2	= 1.196 yd^2
1 hectare (ha)	= 2.4711 acres
1 km^2	= 100 ha = 0.3861 m^2
1 in.^{2}	= 645.16 mm^2
1 yd^2	= 0.8361 m^2
1 acre	= 4840 yd^2 = 4046.86 m^2
1 mile^2	= 640 acres = 2.59 km^2

Water

1 milliliter	= 1 ml = cm^3
1 ml of water	= 1 g
1 L = 1000 ml	= 1000 cm^3
1 L of	= 1 kg

The specific gravity of water = 1.0

Temperature Conversions

°C	°F	°K	°C	°F	°K
−40	−40.0	233	−10	14.0	263
−39	−38.2	234	−9	15.8	264
−38	−36.4	235	−8	17.6	265
−37	−34.6	236	−7	19.4	266
−36	−32.8	237	−6	21.2	267
−35	−31.0	238	−5	21.2	268
−34	−29.2	239	−4	24.8	269
−33	−27.4	240	−3	26.6	270
−32	−25.6	241	−2	28.4	271
−31	−23.8	242	−1	30.2	272
−30	−22.0	243	0	32.0	273
−29	−20.2	244	1	33.8	274
−28	−18.4	245	2	35.6	275
−27	−16.6	246	3	37.4	276
−26	−14.8	247	4	39.2	277
−25	−13.0	248	5	41.0	278
−24	−11.2	249	6	42.8	279
−23	−9.4	250	7	44.6	280
−22	−7.6	251	8	46.4	281
−21	−5.8	252	9	48.2	282
−20	−4.0	253	10	50.0	283
−19	−2.2	254	11	51.8	284
−18	−0.4	255	12	53.6	285
−17	1.4	256	13	55.4	286
−16	3.2	257	14	57.2	287
−15	5.0	258	15	59.0	288
−14	6.8	259	16	60.8	289
−13	8.6	260	17	62.6	290
−12	10.4	261	18	64.4	291
−11	12.2	262	19	66.2	292

°C	°F	°K	°C	°F	°K
20	68.0	293	51	123.8	324
21	69.8	294	52	125.6	325
22	71.6	295	53	127.4	326
23	73.4	296	54	129.2	327
24	75.2	297	55	131.0	328
25	77.0	298	56	132.8	329
26	78.8	299	57	134.6	330
27	80.6	300	58	136.4	331
28	82.4	301	59	138.2	332
29	84.2	302	60	140.0	333
30	86.0	304	61	141.8	334
31	87.8	305	62	143.6	335
32	89.6	305	63	145.4	336
33	91.4	306	64	147.2	337
34	93.2	307	65	149.0	338
35	95.0	308	66	150.8	339
36	96.8	309	67	152.6	340
37	98.6	310	68	154.4	341
38	100.4	311	69	156.2	342
39	102.2	312	70	158.0	343
40	104.0	313	71	159.8	344
41	105.8	314	72	161.6	345
42	107.6	315	73	163.4	346
43	109.4	316	74	165.2	347
44	111.2	317	75	167.0	348
45	113.0	318	76	168.8	349
46	114.8	319	77	170.6	350
47	116.6	320	78	172.4	351
48	118.4	321	79	174.2	352
49	120.2	322	80	176.0	353
50	122.0	323	81	177.8	354

°C	°F	°K	°C	°F	°K
82	179.6	355	94	201.2	367
83	181.4	356	95	203.0	368
84	183.2	357	96	204.8	369
85	185.0	358	97	206.6	370
86	186.8	359	98	208.4	371
87	188.6	360	99	210.2	372
88	190.4	361	100	212.0	373
89	192.2	362	101	213.8	374
90	194.0	363	102	215.6	375
91	195.8	364	103	217.4	376
92	197.6	365	104	219.2	377
93	199.4	366	105	221.0	378

Temperature Conversion Equations

from Fahrenheit to Celsius: $°C = (°F - 32) \times 5/9$
from Celsius to Fahrenheit: $°F = (9/5 \times °C) + 32$
from Celsius to Kelvin: $°K = °C + 273$
from Kelvin to Celsius: $°C = °K - 273$
from Fahrenheit to Kelvin: $°K = (°F - 32) \times 9/5 + 273$
from Kelvin to Fahrenheit: $°F = 9/5 (°K - 273) + 32$

Rectal Temperatures of Common Species

Species	°F	°C
Horse	100.5	38.0
Cow	101.5	38.5
Sheep	103.0	39.5
Goat	102.0	39.0
Pig	102.0	39.0
Dog	102.0	39.0
Cat	101.5	38.5
Rabbit	102.5	39.3

Conversion Factors

Length
1 km = 1000 m
1 hm = 100 m
1 Dm or dam = 10 m
1 meter (m)
1 dm = 0.1 m
1 cm = 0.01 m
1 mm = 0.001 m
1 μm = 0.000001 m
1 nm = 0.000000001 m

Volume
1 kl = 1000 L
1 hl = 100 L
1 Dl = 10 L
1 liter (L) = 1000 ml = 10 dl
1 dl = 0.1 L
1 cl = 0.01 L
1 ml = 0.001 L
1 uL = 0.000,001 L

Weight
1 kg = 1000 g
1 hg = 100 g
1 Dg = 10 g
1 gram (g)
1 dg = 0.1 g
1 cg = 0.01 g
1 mg = 0.001 g
1 μg = 1 mcg = 0.000001 g
1 ng = 0.000000001 g

grams × 0.000001 = micrograms
grams × 0.001 = milligrams
grams × 0.01 = centigrams
grams × 0.1 = decigrams
grams × 1 = grams
grams × 10 = dekagrams
grams × 100 = hectograms

grams × 1000 = kilograms
grams × 1,000,000 = megagrams
grams × 1,000,000,000 = gigagrams

micrometers × 1,000,000 = meters
millimeters × 1000 = meters
centimeters × 100 = meters
decimeters × 10 = meters
meters × 1 = meters
dekameters × 0.1 = meters
hectometers × 0.01 = meters
kilometers × 0.001 = meters

Apothecary Measures
Fluid Measures
60 minims = 1 fluid drachm = fluidrachm
8 fluidrachm = 1 fluid ounce
16 fluid ounces = 1 pint
2 pints = 1 quart = 32 ounces
8 pints = 4 quarts = 1 gallon

Weight Measures
1 grain = 65 mg
20 grains = 1 scruple
3 scruples = 60 grains = 1 drachm
8 drachams = 480 grains = 1 ounce
12 ounces = 5,760 grains = 1 pound

Avoirdupois Measures
Fluid Measures
1 ounce = 29.37 ml
8 ounces = 1 cup = 237 ml
2 cups = 1 pint = 473 ml
2 pints = 1 quart = 946 ml
4 quarts = 1 gallon = 3,785 ml

Weight
1 ounce = 28.35 grams
16 ounces = 1 pound = 454 grams

Length
1 inch = 2.54 centimeters
12 inches = 1 foot
3 feet = 1 yard
5,285 feet = 1 mile

Approximate Household Measures
1 drop = 1/20 ml = 0.05 ml
1 teaspoon (tsp) = 5 ml
1 dessert spoon = 8 ml
1 tablespoon (Tbs) = 3 tsp = 15 ml
1 ounce (oz) = 2 Tbs = 30 ml (29.56 ml)
1 wineglass = 60 ml
1 cup = 8 oz = 240 ml (237 ml)
1 pint (pt) = 2 cups = 480 ml (473 ml)
1 quart = 960 ml (946 ml)
1 gallon (gal) = 4 qt = 3785 ml

Conversion Chart
It is common in practice to encounter situations in which a dose is listed in one system of measurement and a drug is provided in a composition that lists a different system of measurement. To simplify conversions between different systems of measurement, a chart has been designed that allows most common conversions to be performed using simple multiplications. For example, to convert 5 liters to quarts, multiply by the conversion factor 1.507 listed in the chart. Thus, 5 L × 1.507 = 7.535 quarts.

Conversion Chart

To Convert from	to	Multiply by
AREA		
square millimeters (ml²)	square inches (in.²)	0.0016
	square centimeters (cm²)	0.01
square centimeters (cm²)	square inches (in.²)	0.1550
	square feet (ft²)	0.001076
	square millimeters (m²)	100
	square meters (m²)	0.0001
square inches (in.²)	square millimeters (m²)	645.16
	square centimeters (cm²)	6.4516
	square feet (ft²)	0.0069
square feet (ft²)	square centimeters (cm²)	929
	square inches (in.²)	144
	square yards (yd²)	0.1111
	square meters (m²)	0.092903
centares	square meters (m²)	1
VOLUME		
cubic centimeters (cm³)	cubic inches (in.³)	0.0610
	cubic feet (ft³)	3.531×10^{-5}
	pints (pt)	0.0021
	quarts (qt)	0.0011
	liters (L)	0.001
	gallons (gal)	2.642×10^{-4}
cubic inches (in.³)	cubic feet (ft³)	0.0005787
	cubic centimeters (cm³)	16.39
	ounces (oz)	0.5541
	pints (pt)	0.0346
	quarts (qt)	0.0173
	gallons (gal)	0.004329
	drams*	4.4329
	milliliters (ml)	16.3866
	liters (L)	0.01639
cubic feet (ft³)	cubic inches (in.³)	1728
	pints (pt)	59.84
	quarts (qt)	29.92
	gallons (gal)	7.4805
	liters (L)	28.32

Drams are also referred to as fluid dram (fl dr) when a volume is measured or dram if a mass is measured.

To Convert from	to	Multiply by
cubic yards	pints (pt)	1616
(yd³)	quarts (qt)	807.9
	gallons (gal)	202
	liters (L)	764.5
cubic meters	pints (pt)	2113
(m³)	quarts (qt)	1057
	gallons (gal)	264.2
	liters (L)	1000
bushel	liters (L)	35.239
cup	tablespoon (Tbs)	16
	ounces (oz)	8
	pint (pt)	0.5
	milliliters (ml)	237
drops	milliliters (ml)	0.05
fluid dram	minims	60
(fl dr)	milliliters (ml)	3.697
gallon (US)	ounces (oz)	128
(gal)	pints (pt)	8
	quarts (qt)	4
	cubic inches (in.³)	231
	cubic feet (ft³)	0.1337
	milliliters (ml)	3785
	liters (L)	3.785
	cubic centimeter (cm³)	3785
	cubic meters (m³)	0.0038
	imperial gallons	0.8327
gallon (imperial)	gallons, US (gal)	1.2009
gallon (water)	pounds water (lb)	8.34
liters	ounces	33.815
(L)	pints	2.113
	quarts	1.507
	gallon (US)	0.2642
	imperial gallons	0.22
	cubic inches	61.02
	cubic feet	0.0353
	drams	270.52
	deciliters	10
	centiliters	100

To Convert from	to	Multiply by
VOLUME (cont.)		
liters	milliliters	1000
	cubic centimeters	1000
	microliters	1,000,000
	cubic decimeter	1
	cubic meters	0.001
microliters	liters	0.000001
	milliliters	0.001
milliliters	drops	20
(ml)	ounces	0.03381
	quarts	0.00106
	gallons	0.0002642
	cubic inches	0.061
	drams	0.2705
	minims	16.23
	liters	0.001
	microliters	1000
minims	drams	0.01667
	milliliters	0.0616
ounces (fluid)	cups	0.125
	pints	0.0625
	quarts	0.03125
	gallons	0.00781
	cubic inches	1.8047
ounces (apothecary)	drams	8
	milliliters	29.37
ounces (avoirdupois)	drams	16
	milliliters	29.573
	liters	0.02957
pints	ounces	16
	quarts	0.5
	gallons	0.125
	milliliters	473
	liters	0.47
quarts	ounces	32
	pints	2
	gallons	0.25
	cubic inches	57.75
	drams	256
	milliliters	946.332

To Convert from	to	Multiply by
quarts	liters	0.9463
tablespoons	teaspoons	3
	milliliters	15
teaspoons	milliliters	5

VOLUME RATES

cubic feet/minute	gallons/second (gal/sec)	0.1247
	gallons/minute (gal/min)	448.831
	liters/second (L/sec)	0.4719
cubic yards/minute	cubic feet/second (ft³/sec)	0.45
	gallons/second (gal/sec)	3.367
	liters/second (L/sec)	12.74
cubic feet/hour	liter/minute (L/min)	0.472
liters/minute	cubic feet/hour	2.12
milliliters/minute	cubic feet/hour	0.00212

MASS

centigrams	grams	0.01
decigrams	grams	0.1
dekagrams	grams	10
drams*	ounces (avoirdupois)	16
	ounces (apothecary)	8
	grains (avoirdupois)	27.34
	grains (apothecary)	60
grain	ounces	0.00208
	pounds	0.0001429
	grams	0.0648
	milligrams	64.5
	kilograms	0.000065
grams	ounces	0.0353
	grains	15.432
	pounds	0.002205
	ounces (troy)	0.03215
	dynes	980.7
	milligrams	1000
	micrograms	1,000,000
	kilograms	0.001
hectograms	grams	100

To Convert from	to	Multiply by
MASS (cont.)		
kilograms	ounces	32.15
	pounds	2.2046
	grams	1000
	grains	15432.358
	dynes	980665
megagrams	grams	1,000,000
	dynes	980665
micrograms	grams	0.000001
	milligrams	0.001
milligrams	grain	0.0154
	grams	0.001
	micrograms	1000
millimoles	moles	0.001
ounces	ounces (troy)	0.9115
	pounds (avoirdupois)	0.0625
	kilograms	0.0311
ounce (apothecary)	grams	31.1
	grains	480
	drams*	8
ounce (avoirdupois)	grams	28.35
	grains	437.5
	drams	16
pounds	pounds (troy)	1.2153
	hundred weight	100
	drams*	256
pounds (apothecary)	grains	5760
pounds (avoirdupois)	ounces	16
	grains	7000
	grams	454
	kilograms	0.45354
scrupple	grains	20
	grams	1.296
LENGTH AND DISTANCE		
centimeters	inches	0.3937
	feet	0.03281
	yards	0.0109
	millimeters	10
	meters	0.01
decimeter	meters	0.1

To Convert from	to	Multiply by
	inches	4
degrees (angle)	seconds	3600
	radians	0.0174
	minutes	60
dekameter	meters	10
fathom	feet	6
feet	yards	0.3333
	centimeters	30.48
	millimeters	304.8
	meters	0.3048
meters	micrometers	0.001
	millimeters	0.000001
	centimeters	1000
	decimeters	1000
	dekameters	1
	hectometers	0.001
	kilometers	0.000001
micrometers	millimeters	0.001
	meters	0.000001
	millimicrons	1000
	nanometers	1000
microns	micrometers	1
	millimeters	0.001
	meters	0.000001
	millimicrons	1000
	nanometers	1000
millimeter	inches	0.03937
	feet	0.00328
	yards	0.0011
	micron	1000
	micrometers	1000
	centimeters	0.1
	meters	0.001
millimicrons	nanometers	1
	micrometers	0.001
	microns	0.001
nanometers	millimicrons	1
	micrometers	0.001
	microns	0.001
quadrants	radians	1.571

To Convert from	to	Multiply by
radians	quadrants	0.637
	degrees	57.3
	minutes	3438
seconds (angle)	radians	4.841×10^{-6}
	grams	454
	kilograms	0.45354
	grains	20
	grams	1.296

Constants

Speed of light	c	29979250	108 msec-1
Electron charge	e	1.6021917	10-19 C
Avogadro number	N	6.022169	1026 kmole-1
Electron mass (rest)	me	9.109558	10-31 kg
	me	5.485930	10-4 amu
Proton mass (rest)	Mp	1.672614	10-27 kg
	Mp	1.00727661	amu
Neutron mass (rest)	Mn	1.674920	10-27 kg
	Mn	1.00866520	amu
Atomic mass unit	amu	1.660531	10-27 kg
Charge to mass ratio	e/me	1.7588028	1011 Ckg-1
Planck constant	h	6.626196	10-34 J-sec
Rydberg constant	Roo	1.09737312	107 m-1
Gas constant	Ro	8.31434	103 J-kmole-1 K-1
Boltzmann constant	k	1.380622	10-23 JK-1
Gravitational constant	G	6.6732	10-11N-m² kg-2
Bohr magneton	uB	9.274096	10-24 JT-1
Electron magnetic moment	ue	9.284851	10-24 JT-1
Proton magnetic moment	up	1.4106203	10-26 JT-1
Compton wavelength (electron)		2.4263096	10-12 m
Compton wavelength (proton)		1.3214409	10-15 m
Compton wavelength (neutron)		1.3196217	10-15 m
Faraday constant	F	9.648670	107 Ck mole-1

electron mass	0.00055
proton mass	1.0073
neutron mass	1.0087

Other Conversions

% alcohol × 2 = proof
calorie × 1000 = Calories (kilocalories, Kcal)
calorie (kilocalories) × 4,184 = joules
calorie × 3.468 × 10^{-3} = BTU
calorie × 4.184 = joules
joules × 0.2386 = Calories (kilocalories , Kcal)
joules × 9.478 × 10^{-4} = BTU
kilowatt × 1.34 = horsepower
liters × M = moles
milliliters × M = millimoles

Gallons to Pounds
Multiply the specific gravity of the liquid by 8.33 (weight of 1 gallon of water in pounds); and then multiply by the number of gallons.

Grams to Milliliters
Divide the number of grams by the specific gravity.

Milliliters to Grams
Multiply the number of milliliters by the specific gravity.

Milliliters to Ounces (weight)
Multiply the specific gravity by the number of milliliters and divide by 28.35 grams (the number of grams in 1 ounce).

Milliliters to Pounds
Multiply the number of milliliters by the specific gravity and divide by 454 grams (the number of grams in 1 pound).

Ounces (weight) to Milliliters

Multiply the number of ounces by 28.35 grams (the number of grams in 1 ounce) and divide by the specific gravity.

Pounds to Gallons

Multiply the specific gravity by 8.33 pounds per gallon and divide by the number of pounds.

Pounds to Milliliters

Multiply the number of pounds by 454 grams and divide by the specific gravity.

Answers to Practice Problems

Chapter 1
Math Basics
Converting Fractions
to Decimals
1. 0.5
2. ≈ 0.44
3. ≈ 0.429
4. 0.9
5. ≈ 0.067
6. 0.4
7. 0.67
8. 0.625
9. 0.42
10. 0.75

Fractions and Decimals
11. 2.56, 8.84, 0.2695, 45.2
12. 0.94, 0.007, 0.1633, ≈ 3.33
13. 12.82, 1.2, 24.7665, 1.8571
14. 0.17, 4.97, 0.006,
    ≈ 83.83
15. 0.021, 0.12, 0.002, 1.545
16. 4.6, 1.2, 4.08, 3.4
17. 0.022, 0.002, 0.0004, 3
18. 1.7, 2.34, 0.66, ≈ 3.21
19. 3.54, 11.13, 0.152, 4.6254
20. 8.84, 6.76, 16.578, ≈ 57.3

Ratios and Proportions
21. 100 ml
22. 40 ml
23. 6 ml
24. 20 min
25. 0.16%

Temperature
26. 69.8 °F
27. 0 °C
28. 100 °C
29. 48.2 °F
30. 246 °K

Units
31. 0.25 mg
32. 136 U
33. 1 ml
34. 0.04 ml
35. 1 ml

Volume
36. 57,881.25 cm³ (ml) = 15.29 gal
37. 8 ft³ = 59.85 gal
38. 27 ft³ = 202 gal

Moles
39. 0.17 moles
40. 149.1 g
41. 3.4 moles
42. 13.3 moles
43. 210.3 moles

Millimoles
44. 227.9 mmoles
45. 701 mg = 0.7 g
46. 26,277.8 mmoles
47. 0.2997 ≈ 3
48. 13.5 mmoles

Milliequivalents
49. 19.25 ml
50. 145.7 ml
51. 7.5 ml
52. 10 ml
53. 9.82 ml

Milliosmoles
54. 154 mOsm
55. 1028.6 mOsm/L
56. 309.5 mOsm/L
57. 4,000 mOsm/L
58. 2.04 mOsm/ml
    = 2040 mOsm/L

Molarity
59. 1.54 M
60. 0.016 M
61. 3.94 ≈ 4 M
62. 0.015 M
63. 0.006 M

Normality
64. 12 N
65. 83.3 ml
66. 4 N
67. 6 N
68. 2 N

Body Surface Area
69. 62 mg
70. 0.8 mg
71. 23.3
72. 2.14 mg
73. 3400 units

Dropper Calibration
74. 37.5 drops
75. 10 drops
76. 10 drops
77. 30 drops
78. 0.8 ml

Density
79. 35 lb
80. 20.8 lb
81. 6.66 lb
82. 20 lb
83. 0.58

Dilutions
84. 40 ml
85. 60 ml
86. 0.0465 mEq/ml
87. 0.1 L = 100 ml
88. 10 gallons

Drug Dosing
89. 0.2 mg tablet
90. 19.25 ml
91. 1769 mg
92. 1 g
93. 1250 mg

I.V. Drips and Solutions
94. 3.4 ml/hr
95. 8 gtt/min
96. 11.9 ≈ 12 hrs
97. 100 ml/hr
98. 2.5 ml
99. 144 ml
100. 1 mg/ml

ppm
101. 5,000 ppm
102. 0.3785 g
103. 5 ml
104. 11.4 ≈ 11.5 of 500 mg tablets
    22.7 ≈ 23 of 250 mg tablets
105. 164,000 ppm

Percentage
106. 0.41%
107. 250 mg
108. 0.075%
109. 23.65 g
110. 257 mEq
111. 0.4%
112. 10%
113. 55.5 ml

PNU
114. 0.5 ml
115. 0.1 ml
116. 0.83 ml
    2.5 ml
117. 1 ml
118. 16,700 PNU/ml

Chapter 2
Compounding

Capsules
119. a) 322 mg
    b) 5.152 ≈ 6
    c) 159 mg
120. a) 1.3 ≈ 2
    b) 2,489 mg =
       2.489 g
121. a) 3
    b) 5.16 g
122. a) 4.3 ≈ 5
    b) 3,557 mg = 3.557 g

Oral Suspensions
123. 10
124. 3
125. 11.1 ml

Eye Drops
126. 0.875 ml
127. 14.9 mg/ml
128. 2.998%
129. 10 ml
130. 1%

Topical Preparations
131. a) 0.5 mg/ml
    b) 5 mg/ml
    c) 50%
132. 33.11 g
133. 2,530 ml
134. 0.5%
135. a) 0.5%
    b) 202 mcg/ml

Chapter 3
Nutritional Support
BER
136. 1132 Kcal/day
137. 174.87 ≈ 175 Kcal/day
138. 129 Kcal/day
139. 438.6 Kcal/day
140. 91.3 Kcal/day

AER
141. BER = 394 Kcal, AER = 492 Kcal
142. BER = 628 Kcal, AER = 942 Kcal
143. BER = 18.5 Kcal, AER = 27.7 Kcal
144. BER = 737.7 Kcal, AER = 922 Kcal
145. BER = 33 Kcal, AER = 41.8 Kcal

Chapter 4
Toxicology
146. 34.09 mg
147. 5.45 mg to 12 mg
148. 320 ml
149. 1.03 ml or 68.2 mg
150. 3.2ml to 6.4 ml
151. 0.75 mg = 0.125 tab

Selected Protein-Calorie Supplements

Selected Protein-Calorie Supplements

Product (g/dl)	Description	Kcal/ml	mOsm/L	Protein
Clinicare, Feline	Isotonic, low residue	0.92	368	7.0
Clinicare, K9	Isotonic, low residue	0.98	340	5.0
Enrich®	High fiber	1.10	480	4.0
Ensure®	Low residue	1.06	470	3.7
Isocal®	Isotonic, low residue	1.06	270	3.4
Isocal HN®	High nitrogen	1.06	300	4.4
Jevity®	Isotonic, high fiber	1.06	310	4.4
MCT Oil	Medium chain triglycerides (fat)	7.70		—
Osmolite®	Isotonic, low residue	1.06	300	3.7
Osmolite HN®	Isotonic, low residue	1.06	300	4.4
Renal Care, Fel.	Low protein	0.84	260	4.6
Renal Care, K9	Low protein	0.88	250	2.2
Resource®		1.06	470	3.7
Pulmocare	Low residue, high fat	1.50	490	6.3
Reabilan®	Small peptide	1.00	300	3.15
Reabilan HN®	Small peptides and MCT	1.33	490	5.7
Sustacal®	Low residue	1.00	300	4.4
Travasorb Hepatic®	Hepatic diet, high branched chain AA	1.20	300	6.8
Travasorb Renal®	Low residue, electrolyte free, no fat soluble vitamins	1.35	590	2.3
Vital HN®	Elemental diet	1.00	500	4.0
Vivonex TEN®	Elemental diet	1.00	630	3.8

Power
Conversions

If you have a scientific calculator with a y^x key for a number taken to a whole power:

Enter the number, y.
Press the y^x key.
Enter the power, x.
Press equal.

If you do not have a y^x key on your calculator, then multiply y x number of times. For example, 17^3 is 17 × 17 × 17 or 4,913.

To calculate y to a fractional power, for example, to find $y^{0.75}$, first multiply y × y × y. Then, take the sqaure root of the product. Finally, take the sqaure root again. For example, to calculate $4.5^{0.75}$:

4.5 × 4.5 × 4.5 = 91.125

$\sqrt{91.125}$ = 9.545

$\sqrt{9.545}$ = 3.09

Lightning Source UK Ltd.
Milton Keynes UK
27 October 2010

161960UK00001B/27/A